Welcome to the **"Renal Diet Cookbook for Seniors Over 60: 110+ Recipes – A Comprehensive Guide to Managing Renal Health."** This cookbook is dedicated to providing you with delicious, nutritious, and kidney-friendly recipes tailored specifically for seniors aged 60 and above.

As we age, our dietary needs evolve, especially if we are managing kidney health. A renal diet is crucial for individuals with kidney disease or those at risk of developing it, as it helps to manage electrolyte levels, regulate fluid intake, and reduce the workload on the kidneys. This cookbook aims to simplify the process of maintaining a renal-friendly diet by offering a wide variety of recipes that are not only healthy but also enjoyable.

Inside these pages, you will find over 110 recipes that have been carefully crafted with your health and well-being in mind. Whether you are new to a renal diet or have been following one for years, you will discover dishes that are both satisfying and supportive of your kidney health goals.

Each recipe in this book includes clear instructions, nutritional information, and tips to help you navigate the specifics of a renal diet effortlessly. From comforting soups and hearty main dishes to tempting desserts and refreshing beverages, there is something here for every meal and occasion.

In addition to the recipes, this book serves as a comprehensive guide to understanding renal health and the principles of a renal diet. You will find valuable information on key nutrients, portion control, ingredient substitutions, and practical tips for grocery shopping and meal planning.

Our goal is to empower you to take charge of your health through delicious and nourishing food choices. By incorporating these recipes into your daily life, you can support your kidney function, enhance your overall well-being, and enjoy meals that are both beneficial and delightful.

Thank you for embarking on this culinary journey with us. Here's to good health and great flavors!

Warm regards,

Daisy Robinson

1. Scrambled eggs with low•phosphorus cheese

Ingredient:

- 2 large eggs
- 1 tbsp low•fat milk
- 1 oz low•phosphorus cheese (such as cheddar or mozzarella)
- Salt and pepper to taste

Instructions:

1. Crack the eggs into a small bowl and beat them lightly with a fork. Add the milk and whisk until well combined.

2. Spray a small non•stick skillet with cooking spray and heat over medium heat.

3. Pour the egg mixture into the skillet and let it sit for 20•30 seconds to set the bottom.

4. Using a spatula, gently push the cooked egg from the edges into the center, tilting the pan to allow the uncooked egg to flow to the edges.

5. Continue this process, gently folding and stirring the eggs, until they are softly scrambled and no longer runny, about 2•3 minutes.

6. Remove the skillet from the heat and stir in the low•phosphorus cheese until it is melted and well incorporated.

7. Season with salt and pepper to taste.

8. Serve immediately.

This recipe is low in phosphorus, which is important for seniors with kidney disease or on a renal diet. The low•phosphorus cheese helps keep the phosphorus content down. Enjoy!

2. Oatmeal with sliced apples and cinnamon

Ingredient:

- 1/2 cup old·fashioned oats
- 1 cup unsweetened almond milk (or low·fat milk)
- 1 small apple, cored and thinly sliced
- 1/2 tsp ground cinnamon
- 1 tbsp honey (optional)

Instructions:

1. In a small saucepan, combine the oats and almond milk. Bring to a simmer over medium heat, stirring occasionally.

2. Reduce heat to low and continue cooking the oatmeal, stirring frequently, until thickened to your desired consistency, about 5·7 minutes.

3. Remove the oatmeal from heat and stir in the sliced apples and cinnamon.

4. If desired, drizzle with a small amount of honey for added sweetness.

This oatmeal recipe is a great option for seniors on a renal diet for a few reasons:

- Oats are low in phosphorus and potassium, making them a kidney·friendly grain.

- Apples are also low in phosphorus and potassium, providing fiber, vitamins, and natural sweetness.

- Cinnamon adds flavor without adding any additional minerals.

- The almond milk or low·fat milk keeps the recipe low in phosphorus compared to using regular dairy milk.

Enjoy this warm, comforting breakfast that is gentle on the kidneys!

3. Poached eggs on whole wheat toast

Ingredient:

- 2 large eggs
- 2 slices of whole wheat bread
- 1 tsp white vinegar
- Salt and pepper to taste

Instructions:

1. Fill a medium saucepan with 3•4 inches of water and bring to a gentle simmer over medium heat. Add the white vinegar to the water.

2. Crack the eggs one at a time into a small bowl or ramekin. Gently slide the eggs from the bowl into the simmering water.

3. Poach the eggs for 4•5 minutes, until the whites are completely set but the yolks are still runny.

4. While the eggs are poaching, toast the two slices of whole wheat bread.

5. Using a slotted spoon, carefully remove the poached eggs from the water and place them on top of the toasted whole wheat bread.

6. Season with a pinch of salt and pepper.

This recipe is a great option for seniors on a renal diet for a few reasons:

- Whole wheat bread is lower in phosphorus compared to white bread.

- Eggs are a high•quality protein source that is gentle on the kidneys.

- Poaching the eggs avoids the added fat and calories of frying or scrambling.

- The dish is simple and easy to prepare, making it a convenient meal for seniors.

Enjoy this nutritious and kidney•friendly breakfast or brunch option!

4. Low·sodium turkey bacon with scrambled egg whites

Ingredient:

• 2 slices low·sodium turkey bacon
• 2 large egg whites
• 1 tbsp low·fat milk
• Salt and pepper to taste

Instructions:
1. In a small non·stick skillet, cook the turkey bacon over medium heat until crispy, about 3·4 minutes per side. Transfer the cooked bacon to a paper towel·lined plate.

2. In a small bowl, whisk together the egg whites and milk until well combined.

3. Spray the same skillet with a small amount of non·stick cooking spray and heat over medium heat.

4. Pour the egg white mixture into the skillet and let it sit for 20·30 seconds to set the bottom.

5. Using a spatula, gently push the cooked egg from the edges into the center, tilting the pan to allow the uncooked egg to flow to the edges.

6. Continue this process, gently folding and stirring the egg whites, until they are softly scrambled and no longer runny, about 2·3 minutes.

7. Remove the skillet from the heat and season the scrambled egg whites with a pinch of salt and pepper. Serve the scrambled egg whites alongside the cooked turkey bacon.

This recipe is a great option for seniors on a renal diet for a few reasons:

• Turkey bacon is lower in sodium compared to traditional pork bacon, making it a better choice for those on a low·sodium diet.

• Egg whites are a high·quality protein source that is gentle on the kidneys.

• The dish is low in phosphorus, an important mineral for those with kidney disease.

Enjoy this simple and nutritious breakfast option!

5. Smoothies with low·potassium fruits (like berries and apples)

Ingredient:

- 1/2 cup frozen blueberries
- 1/2 cup frozen raspberries
- 1 small apple, cored and chopped
- 1 cup unsweetened almond milk
- 1 tbsp honey (optional)

Instructions:

1. In a blender, combine the frozen blueberries, frozen raspberries, chopped apple, and almond milk.

2. Blend on high speed until the mixture is smooth and creamy, about 1·2 minutes.

3. If desired, add the honey and blend again briefly to incorporate.

4. Pour the smoothie into a glass and enjoy immediately.

This smoothie recipe is a great option for seniors on a renal diet for a few reasons:

• Berries and apples are low in potassium, which is important for those with kidney disease.

• Almond milk is low in phosphorus compared to regular dairy milk.

• The honey provides a natural sweetener if desired, without adding a significant amount of minerals.

• Smoothies are an easy and convenient way for seniors to get a nutrient·dense meal or snack.

You can also try variations of this smoothie by using other low·potassium fruits like strawberries, peaches, or pineapple. Just be sure to avoid high·potassium fruits like bananas, oranges, and melons.

Enjoy this refreshing and kidney·friendly smoothie!

6. Grilled chicken salad with mixed greens and olive oil dressing

Ingredient:

- 4 oz boneless, skinless chicken breast
- 2 cups mixed greens (such as spinach, arugula, and romaine)
- 1/4 cup cherry tomatoes, halved
- 1 tbsp olive oil
- 1 tsp balsamic vinegar
- Salt and pepper to taste

Instructions:

1. Preheat a grill or grill pan to medium·high heat.

2. Season the chicken breast with a pinch of salt and pepper.

3. Grill the chicken for 4·5 minutes per side, or until cooked through and no longer pink in the center. Allow the chicken to rest for 5 minutes, then slice or chop it.

4. In a large salad bowl, combine the mixed greens and cherry tomatoes.

5. In a small bowl, whisk together the olive oil and balsamic vinegar to make the dressing.
6. Drizzle the dressing over the salad and toss to coat.

7. Top the salad with the grilled chicken slices.

This salad recipe is a great option for seniors on a renal diet for a few reasons:

- Grilled chicken is a lean protein source that is gentle on the kidneys.

- Mixed greens are low in potassium and phosphorus, making them a kidney·friendly choice.

- The olive oil dressing is low in sodium and provides healthy fats.

- The dish is easy to prepare and can be customized with different types of greens and vegetables.

Enjoy this nutritious and flavorful salad as a main meal or a side dish.

7. Tuna salad with low·sodium mayonnaise on whole wheat bread

Ingredient:

• 5 oz can of water·packed tuna, drained
• 2 tbsp low·sodium mayonnaise
• 1 tbsp finely chopped celery
• 1 tbsp finely chopped onion
• 1 tsp Dijon mustard
• Salt and pepper to taste
• 2 slices of whole wheat bread

Instructions:

1. In a small bowl, combine the drained tuna, low·sodium mayonnaise, chopped celery, chopped onion, and Dijon mustard. Mix well until fully incorporated.

2. Season the tuna salad with a pinch of salt and pepper to taste.

3. Toast the two slices of whole wheat bread.

4. Spread the tuna salad evenly between the two slices of toast.

This tuna salad sandwich is a great option for seniors on a renal diet for a few reasons:

• Tuna is a lean protein source that is low in phosphorus and potassium.

• The low·sodium mayonnaise helps keep the sodium content down, which is important for those with kidney disease.

• Whole wheat bread is lower in phosphorus compared to white bread.

• The addition of celery and onion provides some extra flavor and texture without adding significant amounts of minerals.

This sandwich makes for a quick and easy lunch or light meal that is gentle on the kidneys. You can also serve the tuna salad on a bed of mixed greens for an alternative option.

Enjoy this tasty and kidney·friendly tuna salad sandwich!

8. Vegetable soup with lean beef or chicken

Ingredient:

- 4 cups low•sodium chicken or beef broth
- 1 cup diced carrots
- 1 cup diced celery
- 1 cup diced zucchini
- 1/2 cup diced onion
- 4 oz lean beef or chicken, cubed
- 1 tsp dried thyme
- Salt and pepper to taste

Instructions:

1. In a large pot, bring the low•sodium broth to a simmer over medium heat.

2. Add the diced carrots, celery, zucchini, and onion to the pot. Simmer for 10•15 minutes, or until the vegetables are tender.

3. Add the cubed lean beef or chicken to the pot and continue simmering for an additional 5•7 minutes, or until the meat is cooked through.

4. Stir in the dried thyme and season with a pinch of salt and pepper to taste.

5. Ladle the vegetable soup into bowls and serve hot.

This vegetable soup recipe is a great option for seniors on a renal diet for a few reasons:

- The low•sodium broth helps keep the sodium content down, which is important for those with kidney disease.

- The vegetables, such as carrots, celery, and zucchini, are low in potassium and phosphorus.

- The lean beef or chicken provides a source of protein that is gentle on the kidneys.

- The simple seasoning with thyme adds flavor without adding significant amounts of minerals.

This soup can be a satisfying and nutritious meal on its own, or it can be served with a small portion of whole grain bread or crackers.

9. Quinoa salad with cucumber, tomatoes, and lemon dressing

Ingredient:

- 1 cup cooked quinoa, cooled
- 1 cup diced cucumber
- 1 cup cherry tomatoes, halved
- 2 tbsp chopped fresh parsley
- 2 tbsp olive oil
- 1 tbsp lemon juice
- 1 tsp Dijon mustard
- Salt and pepper to taste

Instructions:

1. In a large bowl, combine the cooked and cooled quinoa, diced cucumber, halved cherry tomatoes, and chopped parsley. Mix well.

2. In a small bowl, whisk together the olive oil, lemon juice, and Dijon mustard to make the dressing.

3. Pour the dressing over the quinoa salad and toss gently to coat.

4. Season the salad with a pinch of salt and pepper to taste. Serve chilled or at room temperature.

This quinoa salad is a great option for seniors on a renal diet for a few reasons:

- Quinoa is a whole grain that is low in phosphorus and potassium, making it a kidney·friendly choice.

- Cucumbers and tomatoes are also low in these minerals, providing a nutrient·dense base for the salad.

- The lemon dressing is low in sodium and provides a bright, refreshing flavor.

- The dish is easy to prepare and can be made in advance, making it a convenient option for seniors.

This salad can be enjoyed as a light main course or a side dish. It's also a great option for meal prepping and can be stored in the refrigerator for up to 3·4 days.

10. Baked Fish with steamed vegetables

Ingredient:

• 4 (4 oz) white fish fillets (such as tilapia, cod, or halibut)
• 1 tbsp olive oil
• 1 tsp lemon pepper seasoning
• 1 cup broccoli florets
• 1 cup cauliflower florets
• 1 cup sliced zucchini
• 2 tbsp low·sodium vegetable broth

Instructions:
1. Preheat your oven to 400°F (200°C).

2. Place the fish fillets in a baking dish and drizzle with the olive oil. Sprinkle the lemon pepper seasoning over the top.

3. Bake the fish in the preheated oven for 12·15 minutes, or until it flakes easily with a fork.
4. While the fish is baking, prepare the steamed vegetables. In a large steamer basket, combine the broccoli florets, cauliflower florets, and sliced zucchini.

5. Place the steamer basket over a pot of simmering water and steam the vegetables for 5·7 minutes, or until they are tender·crisp.

6. Transfer the steamed vegetables to a bowl and toss with the low·sodium vegetable broth. Serve the baked fish fillets alongside the steamed vegetables.

This baked fish with steamed vegetables is a great option for seniors on a renal diet for a few reasons:

• White fish, such as tilapia, cod, or halibut, are low in phosphorus and potassium, making them a kidney·friendly protein source.

• The steamed vegetables, including broccoli, cauliflower, and zucchini, are also low in these minerals, providing a nutrient·dense side dish.

• The simple seasoning with lemon pepper adds flavor without adding significant amounts of sodium or other minerals. The dish is easy to prepare and can be a complete, balanced meal.

11. Baked salmon with dill sauce

Ingredient:

- 4 (4 oz) salmon fillets
- 1 tbsp olive oil
- Salt and pepper to taste
- 1/4 cup plain Greek yogurt
- 2 tbsp chopped fresh dill
- 1 tbsp lemon juice
- 1 tsp Dijon mustard
- 1 garlic clove, minced

Instructions:

1. Preheat your oven to 400°F (200°C).

2. Place the salmon fillets on a baking sheet lined with parchment paper. Drizzle the fillets with the olive oil and season with salt and pepper.

3. Bake the salmon in the preheated oven for 12•15 minutes, or until it flakes easily with a fork.

4. While the salmon is baking, prepare the dill sauce. In a small bowl, combine the Greek yogurt, chopped dill, lemon juice, Dijon mustard, and minced garlic. Stir until well mixed.

5. Serve the baked salmon fillets warm, with the dill sauce spooned over the top.

This baked salmon with dill sauce is a great option for seniors on a renal diet for a few reasons:

- Salmon is a fatty fish that is high in omega•3 fatty acids, which are beneficial for heart and kidney health.

- The dill sauce is low in phosphorus and potassium, providing a flavorful topping without adding significant amounts of these minerals.

- The dish is easy to prepare and can be a quick and nutritious meal.

You can serve the salmon with a side of steamed or roasted low•potassium vegetables, such as broccoli, cauliflower, or zucchini, for a complete and kidney•friendly meal.

Enjoy this delicious and healthy baked salmon with dill sauce!

12. Stir·fried tofu with low·sodium soy sauce and vegetables

Ingredient:
- 1 block (14 oz) firm or extra·firm tofu, cubed
- 2 tbsp low·sodium soy sauce
- 1 tbsp rice vinegar
- 1 tsp sesame oil
- 1 tbsp olive oil
- 2 cups mixed vegetables (such as broccoli, carrots, snow peas, and bell peppers), chopped
- 2 cloves garlic, minced
- 1 tsp grated fresh ginger
- Salt and pepper to taste

Instructions:

1. In a small bowl, combine the low·sodium soy sauce, rice vinegar, and sesame oil. Set aside.

2. Heat the olive oil in a large skillet or wok over medium·high heat.

3. Add the cubed tofu to the skillet and stir·fry for 3·4 minutes, or until lightly browned on all sides. Transfer the tofu to a plate and set aside.

4. Add the chopped mixed vegetables, minced garlic, and grated ginger to the skillet. Stir·fry for 5·7 minutes, or until the vegetables are tender·crisp.

5. Return the tofu to the skillet and pour in the soy sauce mixture. Toss everything together and cook for an additional 2·3 minutes, or until the sauce has thickened slightly.

6. Season the stir·fry with a pinch of salt and pepper to taste. Serve the stir·fried tofu and vegetables over a bed of steamed brown rice or quinoa.

This stir·fried tofu dish is a great option for seniors on a renal diet for a few reasons:
- Tofu is a plant·based protein source that is low in phosphorus and potassium.
- The low·sodium soy sauce helps keep the sodium content down, which is important for those with kidney disease.
- The mixed vegetables, such as broccoli, carrots, and bell peppers, are also low in these minerals.
- The dish is easy to prepare and can be a complete, balanced meal when served with a whole grain like brown rice or quinoa.

13. Roast turkey breast with green beans

Ingredient:

- 2 lb boneless, skinless turkey breast
- 1 tsp dried thyme
- 1 tsp garlic powder
- Salt and pepper to taste
- 1 lb fresh green beans, trimmed
- 2 tbsp olive oil
- 1 tbsp lemon juice

Instructions:

1. Preheat your oven to 375°F (190°C).

2. Place the turkey breast in a baking dish and season it with the dried thyme, garlic powder, salt, and pepper.

3. Roast the turkey breast in the preheated oven for 45·60 minutes, or until it reaches an internal temperature of 165°F (74°C).

4. While the turkey is roasting, prepare the green beans. Bring a large pot of water to a boil. Add the trimmed green beans and blanch for 3·4 minutes, until they are tender·crisp.

5. Drain the green beans and transfer them to a bowl. Toss the green beans with the olive oil and lemon juice. Season with a pinch of salt and pepper.

6. Once the turkey breast is cooked, let it rest for 5·10 minutes before slicing. Serve the sliced turkey breast alongside the lemon·garlic green beans.

This roast turkey breast with green beans is a great option for seniors on a renal diet for a few reasons:

- Turkey breast is a lean protein source that is gentle on the kidneys.

- Green beans are low in potassium and phosphorus, making them a kidney·friendly vegetable.

- The simple seasoning with thyme, garlic, and lemon adds flavor without adding significant amounts of minerals. The dish is easy to prepare and can be a complete, balanced meal.

14. Beef stew with low·potassium vegetables (like carrots and green beans)

Ingredient:

- 1 lb lean beef stew meat, cubed
- 2 cups low·sodium beef broth
- 1 cup diced carrots
- 1 cup diced green beans
- 1 cup diced celery
- 1 onion, diced
- 2 cloves garlic, minced
- 1 tsp dried thyme
- 1 bay leaf
- Salt and pepper to taste

Instructions:

1. In a large pot or Dutch oven, brown the beef stew meat over medium·high heat until it's no longer pink, about 5·7 minutes.

2. Add the low·sodium beef broth, diced carrots, green beans, celery, onion, garlic, dried thyme, and bay leaf. Stir to combine.

3. Bring the stew to a boil, then reduce the heat to low, cover, and simmer for 45·60 minutes, or until the beef and vegetables are tender. Remove the bay leaf and season the stew with salt and pepper to taste.

This beef stew is a great option for seniors on a renal diet for a few reasons:

- Lean beef is a good source of protein that is gentle on the kidneys.

- Carrots and green beans are low in potassium, making them kidney·friendly vegetables.

- Celery and onion add flavor without contributing significant amounts of minerals.

- The low·sodium beef broth helps keep the sodium content down.

- The stew is a one·pot meal that is easy to prepare and can be a comforting, nutritious option.

You can serve the beef stew on its own or with a small portion of whole wheat bread or rolls. Enjoy this delicious and kidney·friendly meal!

15. Eggplant parmesan with whole wheat pasta

Ingredient:

- 1 medium eggplant, sliced into 1/2•inch thick rounds
- 1 cup whole wheat breadcrumbs
- 1/4 cup grated Parmesan cheese
- 2 large eggs, beaten
- 2 cups low•sodium marinara sauce
- 1 cup shredded low•fat mozzarella cheese
- 8 oz whole wheat pasta, cooked according to package instructions

Instructions:

1. Preheat your oven to 375°F (190°C). Line a baking sheet with parchment paper.

2. In a shallow bowl, combine the whole wheat breadcrumbs and grated Parmesan cheese.

3. Dip the eggplant slices into the beaten eggs, then coat them in the breadcrumb mixture, pressing gently to adhere.

4. Arrange the breaded eggplant slices in a single layer on the prepared baking sheet.

5. Bake the eggplant for 20•25 minutes, flipping halfway, until golden brown and tender.

6. Spread 1 cup of the low•sodium marinara sauce in the bottom of a baking dish. Arrange the baked eggplant slices in a single layer over the sauce.

7. Top the eggplant with the remaining 1 cup of marinara sauce and the shredded mozzarella cheese.

8. Bake the eggplant parmesan for an additional 15•20 minutes, or until the cheese is melted and bubbly. Serve the eggplant parmesan over the cooked whole wheat pasta.

This eggplant parmesan dish is a great option for seniors on a renal diet for a few reasons:

- Eggplant is low in potassium and phosphorus, making it a kidney•friendly vegetable.
- Whole wheat breadcrumbs and pasta are lower in phosphorus compared to their refined counterparts.
- The low•sodium marinara sauce helps keep the sodium content down.
- The dish provides a good source of protein from the Parmesan and mozzarella cheeses.

16. Steamed asparagus with lemon

Ingredient:

• 1 lb fresh asparagus, trimmed
• 1 tbsp lemon juice
• 1 tsp olive oil
• Salt and pepper to taste

Instructions:
1. Fill a medium saucepan with about 1 inch of water and bring it to a boil over high heat.

2. Place the trimmed asparagus spears in a steamer basket and carefully lower the basket into the boiling water.

3. Steam the asparagus for 5•7 minutes, or until it is tender•crisp.

4. Remove the steamed asparagus from the heat and transfer it to a serving dish.

5. Drizzle the lemon juice and olive oil over the asparagus and gently toss to coat.

6. Season the asparagus with a pinch of salt and pepper to taste. Serve the steamed asparagus with lemon immediately.

This steamed asparagus with lemon is a great option to support a renal diet for seniors over 60 for a few reasons:

• Asparagus is low in potassium and phosphorus, making it a kidney•friendly vegetable.

• Lemon juice adds a bright, refreshing flavor without adding any significant amounts of minerals.

• The simple preparation method of steaming preserves the nutrients in the asparagus.

• The dish is easy to prepare and can be a quick, healthy side dish.

Asparagus is also a good source of fiber, vitamins, and antioxidants, which can be beneficial for overall health in seniors.

Enjoy this delicious and nutritious steamed asparagus with lemon!

17. Mashed cauliflower with low•fat milk

Ingredient:

- 1 head of cauliflower, cut into florets
- 1/4 cup low•fat milk
- 1 tbsp unsalted butter
- Salt and pepper to taste

Instructions:

1. In a large pot, bring a few inches of water to a boil. Add the cauliflower florets, cover, and steam for 10•12 minutes, or until the cauliflower is very tender.

2. Drain the cooked cauliflower and transfer it to a food processor or high•powered blender.

3. Add the low•fat milk and unsalted butter to the food processor or blender. Blend the mixture until it is smooth and creamy, scraping down the sides as needed.

4. Season the mashed cauliflower with a pinch of salt and pepper to taste. Serve the mashed cauliflower warm.

This mashed cauliflower with low•fat milk is a great option to support a renal diet for seniors over 60 for a few reasons:

- Cauliflower is a low•potassium, low•phosphorus vegetable, making it a kidney•friendly choice.

- The use of low•fat milk helps keep the dish lower in phosphorus compared to using regular milk.

- The unsalted butter adds a creamy texture without contributing significant amounts of sodium.

- The dish is easy to prepare and can be a versatile side dish or base for other meals.

You can also try adding a sprinkle of grated Parmesan cheese or fresh herbs, such as chives or parsley, to the mashed cauliflower for additional flavor.

Enjoy this delicious and nutritious mashed cauliflower with low•fat milk!

18. Brown rice pilaf with herbs

Ingredient:

- 1 cup uncooked brown rice
- 2 cups low•sodium chicken or vegetable broth
- 1 tbsp olive oil
- 1 onion, diced
- 2 cloves garlic, minced
- 1 tsp dried thyme
- 1 tsp dried parsley
- Salt and pepper to taste

Instructions:

1. In a medium saucepan, bring the low•sodium broth to a boil over high heat.

2. Add the uncooked brown rice, cover, and reduce the heat to low. Simmer for 45•50 minutes, or until the rice is tender and the liquid is absorbed.

3. In a separate skillet, heat the olive oil over medium heat. Add the diced onion and sauté for 3•4 minutes, until translucent.

4. Add the minced garlic, dried thyme, and dried parsley to the skillet. Cook for an additional 1•2 minutes, stirring constantly, until fragrant.

5. Fluff the cooked brown rice with a fork and transfer it to the skillet with the onion and herb mixture. Gently stir to combine.

6. Season the brown rice pilaf with a pinch of salt and pepper to taste. Serve the brown rice pilaf warm.

This brown rice pilaf with herbs is a great option to support a renal diet for seniors over 60 for a few reasons:

- Brown rice is a whole grain that is lower in phosphorus compared to white rice, making it a better choice for those with kidney disease.
- The low•sodium broth helps keep the sodium content down.
- The herbs, such as thyme and parsley, add flavor without contributing significant amounts of minerals.
- The dish is easy to prepare and can be a versatile side dish or base for a main meal.

You can also try adding other low•potassium vegetables, such as diced carrots or zucchini, to the pilaf for additional nutrients and flavor.

19. Steamed broccoli with garlic

Ingredient:

- 1 lb fresh broccoli florets
- 2 tbsp water
- 2 cloves garlic, minced
- 1 tbsp olive oil
- Salt and pepper to taste

Instructions:

1. In a large steamer basket, place the broccoli florets. Pour the 2 tbsp of water into the bottom of the steamer pot.

2. Bring the water to a boil over high heat, then reduce the heat to medium•low, cover, and steam the broccoli for 5•7 minutes, or until it is tender•crisp.

3. In a small skillet, heat the olive oil over medium heat. Add the minced garlic and cook for 1•2 minutes, stirring frequently, until fragrant.

4. Transfer the steamed broccoli to a serving bowl. Drizzle the garlic•infused olive oil over the broccoli and toss to coat.

5. Season the broccoli with a pinch of salt and pepper to taste. Serve the steamed broccoli with garlic immediately.

This steamed broccoli with garlic is a great option to support a renal diet for seniors over 60 for a few reasons:

- Broccoli is a low•potassium, low•phosphorus vegetable, making it a kidney•friendly choice.

- The simple steaming method preserves the nutrients in the broccoli.

- The garlic adds flavor without contributing significant amounts of minerals.

- The dish is easy to prepare and can be a quick, healthy side dish.

You can also try adding a squeeze of lemon juice or a sprinkle of grated Parmesan cheese to the broccoli for additional flavor.

Enjoy this delicious and nutritious steamed broccoli with garlic!

20. Roasted Brussels sprouts with balsamic glaze

Ingredient:

- 1 lb Brussels sprouts, trimmed and halved
- 2 tbsp olive oil
- 1/4 tsp salt
- 1/8 tsp black pepper
- 2 tbsp balsamic vinegar
- 1 tbsp honey

Instructions:

1. Preheat your oven to 400°F (200°C).

2. In a large bowl, toss the trimmed and halved Brussels sprouts with the olive oil, salt, and black pepper until the sprouts are evenly coated.

3. Spread the Brussels sprouts in a single layer on a baking sheet lined with parchment paper.

4. Roast the Brussels sprouts in the preheated oven for 20·25 minutes, or until they are tender and lightly browned, stirring halfway through.

5. In a small saucepan, combine the balsamic vinegar and honey. Bring the mixture to a simmer over medium heat and cook for 2·3 minutes, or until it has thickened slightly to a glaze·like consistency.

6. Remove the roasted Brussels sprouts from the oven and drizzle the balsamic glaze over the top, tossing gently to coat. Serve the roasted Brussels sprouts with balsamic glaze immediately.

This roasted Brussels sprouts dish is a great option to support a renal diet for seniors over 60 for a few reasons:

- Brussels sprouts are low in potassium and phosphorus, making them a kidney·friendly vegetable.

- The balsamic glaze adds a sweet and tangy flavor without contributing significant amounts of minerals.

- The simple roasting method preserves the nutrients in the Brussels sprouts. The dish is easy to prepare and can be a delicious and nutritious side dish.

21. Fresh Fruit salad (using low·potassium fruits)

Ingredient:

- 1 cup diced pineapple
- 1 cup diced strawberries
- 1 cup diced blueberries
- 1 cup diced grapes
- 1 cup diced apples
- 1 tbsp lemon juice

Instructions:

1. In a large bowl, combine the diced pineapple, strawberries, blueberries, grapes, and apples.

2. Drizzle the lemon juice over the fruit and gently toss to coat.

3. Cover the fruit salad and refrigerate for at least 30 minutes to allow the flavors to meld.

4. Serve the chilled fruit salad.

This fresh fruit salad is a great option to support a renal diet for seniors over 60 for a few reasons:

• The fruits used (pineapple, strawberries, blueberries, grapes, and apples) are all relatively low in potassium, making them kidney·friendly choices.

• The lemon juice adds a refreshing flavor without contributing significant amounts of minerals.

• Fruit salads are a great way to incorporate a variety of vitamins, minerals, and antioxidants into the diet.

• The dish is easy to prepare and can be a light, healthy snack or dessert.

You can also try adding other low·potassium fruits, such as raspberries, blackberries, or kiwi, to this salad. Just be sure to avoid high·potassium fruits like bananas, oranges, and melons.

22. Rice cakes with almond butter

Ingredient:

• 2 whole grain rice cakes
• 2 tbsp unsalted almond butter
• 1 tsp honey (optional)

Instructions:

1. Spread the unsalted almond butter evenly over the surface of the two rice cakes.

2. If desired, drizzle a small amount of honey over the almond butter for added sweetness.

3. Serve the rice cakes with almond butter immediately.

This rice cakes with almond butter snack is a great option to support a renal diet for seniors over 60 for a few reasons:

• Whole grain rice cakes are low in phosphorus and potassium, making them a kidney•friendly choice.

• Unsalted almond butter is a good source of protein and healthy fats without adding significant amounts of minerals.

• The honey (if used) provides a natural sweetener without contributing high levels of potassium or phosphorus.

• The snack is easy to prepare and can be a quick, portable option for seniors.

You can also try topping the rice cakes with other low•potassium fruits, such as sliced strawberries or blueberries, for added nutrients and flavor.

Enjoy this simple yet satisfying rice cakes with almond butter snack!

23. Greek yogurt with honey and nuts

Ingredient:

- 1 cup plain, low•fat Greek yogurt
- 1 tbsp honey
- 2 tbsp chopped unsalted nuts (such as almonds or walnuts)

Instructions:

1. In a small bowl, combine the plain, low•fat Greek yogurt and honey. Stir until the honey is fully incorporated.

2. Sprinkle the chopped unsalted nuts over the top of the yogurt.

3. Serve the Greek yogurt with honey and nuts immediately.

This Greek yogurt with honey and nuts is a great option to support a renal diet for seniors over 60 for a few reasons:

- Greek yogurt is a good source of protein that is gentle on the kidneys.

- Honey provides a natural sweetener without contributing significant amounts of minerals.

- Unsalted nuts, such as almonds or walnuts, are a source of healthy fats and nutrients without adding high levels of potassium or phosphorus.

- The dish is easy to prepare and can be a nutritious snack or light dessert.

You can also try adding a sprinkle of cinnamon or a few fresh berries to the yogurt for additional flavor and nutrients.

Enjoy this delicious and kidney•friendly Greek yogurt with honey and nuts!

24. Air•popped popcorn (lightly salted)

Ingredient:

• 1/2 cup unpopped popcorn kernels
• 1/4 tsp salt (or to taste)

Instructions:
1. In an air popper, pop the 1/2 cup of unpopped popcorn kernels according to the manufacturer's instructions.

2. Transfer the freshly popped popcorn to a large bowl.

3. Sprinkle the 1/4 tsp of salt over the popcorn and toss gently to coat.

4. Serve the air•popped, lightly salted popcorn immediately.

This air•popped popcorn with light salt is a great option to support a renal diet for seniors over 60 for a few reasons:

• Popcorn is a whole grain that is low in potassium and phosphorus, making it a kidney•friendly snack.

• Air•popping the popcorn avoids the added oils and fats that can come with microwave or stovetop popping methods.

• The small amount of salt added provides just a touch of flavor without contributing high levels of sodium.

• Popcorn can be a satisfying, crunchy snack that is easy to portion control.

You can also try experimenting with other low•sodium seasonings, such as garlic powder, onion powder, or dried herbs, to add more flavor to the popcorn.

Enjoy this simple and nutritious air•popped popcorn with light salt!

25. Homemade trail mix
with unsalted nuts and dried fruits

Ingredient:

- 1/2 cup unsalted almonds
- 1/2 cup unsalted cashews
- 1/4 cup unsalted pumpkin seeds
- 1/4 cup unsalted sunflower seeds
- 1/4 cup dried cranberries
- 1/4 cup diced dried apricots

Instructions:

1. In a large bowl, combine the unsalted almonds, unsalted cashews, unsalted pumpkin seeds, and unsalted sunflower seeds.

2. Add the dried cranberries and diced dried apricots to the nut mixture and stir to mix well.

3. Transfer the trail mix to an airtight container or resealable bag for storage.

This homemade trail mix is a great option to support a renal diet for seniors over 60 for a few reasons:

• Unsalted nuts, such as almonds and cashews, are a good source of protein and healthy fats without adding significant amounts of sodium, potassium, or phosphorus.

• Pumpkin seeds and sunflower seeds provide additional nutrients without contributing high levels of minerals.

• Dried cranberries and dried apricots are lower in potassium compared to many other dried fruits, making them a better choice for those on a renal diet.

• The trail mix is easy to prepare and can be a convenient, portable snack or addition to a meal.

This homemade trail mix can be enjoyed on its own or as a topping for yogurt, oatmeal, or salads. Portion control is important, as nuts and dried fruits can be high in calories, so it's best to stick to the recommended serving size.

26. Chicken noodle soup (low•sodium broth)

Ingredient:

• 4 cups low•sodium chicken broth
• 1 boneless, skinless chicken breast, diced
• 1 cup diced carrots
• 1 cup diced celery
• 1/2 cup diced onion
• 1 cup whole wheat egg noodles
• 2 tbsp fresh parsley, chopped
• Salt and pepper to taste

Instructions:

1. In a large pot, bring the low•sodium chicken broth to a boil over medium•high heat.

2. Add the diced chicken, carrots, celery, and onion. Reduce heat to medium•low and simmer for 10•15 minutes until the vegetables are tender.

3. Add the whole wheat egg noodles and cook for an additional 8•10 minutes until the noodles are tender.

4. Stir in the fresh parsley and season with a small amount of salt and pepper to taste.

This chicken noodle soup is low in sodium, which is important for a renal diet. The whole wheat noodles provide fiber, and the chicken, vegetables, and broth offer protein, vitamins, and minerals that are beneficial for seniors. Enjoy this comforting and nutritious soup!

27. Minestrone soup with kidney beans

Ingredient:

- 4 cups low•sodium vegetable or chicken broth
- 1 cup diced onions
- 1 cup diced carrots
- 1 cup diced celery
- 2 cloves garlic, minced
- 1 (15 oz) can no•salt•added diced tomatoes
- 1 (15 oz) can no•salt•added kidney beans, rinsed and drained
- 1 cup small whole wheat pasta (such as ditalini or small shells)
- 1 tsp dried oregano
- 1 tsp dried basil
- Salt and pepper to taste
- Grated Parmesan cheese (optional)

Instructions:

1. In a large pot, bring the low•sodium broth to a boil over medium•high heat.

2. Add the onions, carrots, celery, and garlic. Reduce heat to medium•low and simmer for 10 minutes.

3. Stir in the diced tomatoes, kidney beans, whole wheat pasta, oregano, and basil. Simmer for an additional 10•15 minutes until the pasta is tender.

4. Season with a small amount of salt and pepper to taste.

5. Serve hot, optionally topped with a sprinkle of grated Parmesan cheese.

This minestrone soup is packed with fiber, protein, and nutrients from the vegetables, beans, and whole grain pasta. The low•sodium broth and no•salt•added canned goods make it kidney•friendly. It's a comforting and nutritious meal for seniors on a renal diet.

28. Tomato basil soup (low•sodium)

Ingredient:

• 1 tbsp olive oil
• 1 onion, diced
• 2 cloves garlic, minced
• 1 (28 oz) can low•sodium diced tomatoes
• 2 cups low•sodium vegetable broth
• 1/4 cup fresh basil leaves, chopped
• 1 tsp dried oregano
• Salt and pepper to taste

Instructions:
1. In a large pot, heat the olive oil over medium heat. Add the diced onion and sauté for 3•4 minutes, until translucent.

2. Add the minced garlic to the pot and cook for an additional 1•2 minutes, until fragrant.

3. Pour in the can of low•sodium diced tomatoes and the low•sodium vegetable broth. Stir to combine.

4. Bring the soup to a simmer and let it cook for 10•15 minutes, allowing the flavors to meld.

5. Remove the pot from the heat and stir in the chopped fresh basil leaves and dried oregano. Use an immersion blender or regular blender to puree the soup until smooth.

6. Season the low•sodium tomato basil soup with a pinch of salt and pepper to taste. Serve the soup warm.

This low•sodium tomato basil soup is a great option to support a renal diet for seniors over 60 for a few reasons:
• The use of low•sodium diced tomatoes and low•sodium vegetable broth helps keep the sodium content down, which is important for those with kidney disease.
• Fresh basil and dried oregano add flavor without contributing significant amounts of minerals.
• The soup is easy to prepare and can be a comforting, nutrient•dense meal.
• Blending the soup creates a smooth, creamy texture without the need for heavy cream or other high•fat ingredients.

You can serve the low•sodium tomato basil soup on its own or with a small portion of whole grain crackers or a side salad.

29. Split pea soup (without ham)

Ingredient:

- 1 cup dried split peas, rinsed
- 4 cups low•sodium vegetable broth
- 1 onion, diced
- 2 carrots, diced
- 2 celery stalks, diced
- 2 cloves garlic, minced
- 1 tsp dried thyme
- Salt and pepper to taste

Instructions:

1. In a large pot, combine the rinsed split peas and low•sodium vegetable broth. Bring the mixture to a boil over high heat.

2. Reduce the heat to low, cover the pot, and let the split peas simmer for 45•60 minutes, stirring occasionally, until the peas are very soft and starting to break down.

3. Add the diced onion, carrots, celery, and minced garlic to the pot. Continue simmering for an additional 15•20 minutes, or until the vegetables are tender.

4. Stir in the dried thyme and season the soup with a pinch of salt and pepper to taste. Serve the split pea soup hot.

This split pea soup without ham is a great option to support a renal diet for seniors over 60 for a few reasons:

- Split peas are a good source of plant•based protein that is low in phosphorus and potassium.

- The low•sodium vegetable broth helps keep the sodium content down, which is important for those with kidney disease.

- The addition of onions, carrots, and celery provides extra nutrients without contributing high levels of minerals.

- The simple seasoning with thyme adds flavor without adding significant amounts of sodium or other minerals. The soup is easy to prepare and can be a comforting, nutritious meal.

30. Butternut squash soup (low·fat)

Ingredient:

- 1 medium butternut squash, peeled, seeded, and cubed (about 4 cups)
- 1 onion, diced
- 2 cloves garlic, minced
- 4 cups low·sodium chicken or vegetable broth
- 1 cup unsweetened almond milk
- 1 tsp ground cinnamon
- 1/4 tsp ground nutmeg
- Salt and pepper to taste
- Chopped parsley for garnish (optional)

Instructions:

1. In a large pot or Dutch oven, sauté the diced onion in a small amount of oil or broth over medium heat for 5 minutes until translucent.

2. Add the minced garlic and sauté for 1 minute until fragrant.

3. Add the cubed butternut squash and low·sodium broth. Bring to a boil, then reduce heat and simmer for 20·25 minutes, until the squash is very soft.

4. Using an immersion blender, carefully blend the soup until smooth and creamy. Alternatively, you can transfer the soup in batches to a regular blender.

5. Stir in the unsweetened almond milk, cinnamon, and nutmeg. Season with a small amount of salt and pepper to taste.

6. Serve hot, garnished with chopped parsley if desired.

This butternut squash soup is low in fat and sodium, making it a great option for a renal diet. The squash provides fiber, vitamins, and minerals, while the almond milk adds creaminess without excess calories or saturated fat. It's a comforting and nourishing soup for seniors.

31. Whole wheat pasta with marinara sauce

Ingredient:

- 8 oz whole wheat pasta (such as penne or spaghetti)
- 1 tbsp olive oil
- 1 onion, diced
- 3 cloves garlic, minced
- 1 (28 oz) can no·salt·added crushed tomatoes
- 2 tbsp fresh basil, chopped
- 1 tsp dried oregano
- 1/4 tsp black pepper
- Grated Parmesan cheese (optional)

Instructions:

1. Bring a large pot of water to a boil. Cook the whole wheat pasta according to package instructions until al dente. Drain and set aside.

2. In a large skillet, heat the olive oil over medium heat. Add the diced onion and sauté for 5 minutes until translucent.

3. Add the minced garlic and sauté for 1 minute until fragrant.

4. Pour in the no·salt·added crushed tomatoes. Stir in the fresh basil, dried oregano, and black pepper.

5. Simmer the marinara sauce for 10·15 minutes, stirring occasionally, until thickened.

6. Add the cooked whole wheat pasta to the sauce and toss to coat.

7. Serve hot, optionally topped with a sprinkle of grated Parmesan cheese.

This whole wheat pasta dish is a great option for seniors on a renal diet. The whole grains provide fiber, and the low·sodium marinara sauce is kidney·friendly. The vegetables and herbs add flavor without excess sodium. It's a simple, nutritious, and satisfying meal.

32. Pasta primavera with olive oil and vegetables

Ingredient:

• 8 oz whole wheat pasta
• 2 tbsp olive oil
• 1 cup broccoli florets
• 1 cup sliced zucchini
• 1 cup sliced mushrooms
• 1 cup cherry tomatoes, halved
• 2 cloves garlic, minced
• 1 tsp dried basil
• Salt and pepper to taste

Instructions:

1. Bring a large pot of water to a boil. Cook the whole wheat pasta according to the package instructions until al dente. Drain the pasta and set it aside.

2. In a large skillet, heat the olive oil over medium heat. Add the broccoli florets, sliced zucchini, sliced mushrooms, and halved cherry tomatoes. Sauté the vegetables for 5•7 minutes, until they are tender•crisp.

3. Add the minced garlic to the skillet and cook for an additional 1•2 minutes, until fragrant.

4. Add the cooked whole wheat pasta to the skillet with the sautéed vegetables. Toss everything together to combine.

5. Sprinkle the dried basil over the pasta primavera and season with a pinch of salt and pepper to taste. Serve the pasta primavera warm.

This pasta primavera dish with olive oil and vegetables is a great option to support a renal diet for seniors over 60 for a few reasons:

• Whole wheat pasta is lower in phosphorus compared to regular pasta, making it a better choice for those with kidney disease.
• The vegetables, including broccoli, zucchini, mushrooms, and tomatoes, are low in potassium and phosphorus.
• Olive oil provides a source of healthy fats without contributing significant amounts of minerals.
• The simple seasoning with basil adds flavor without adding high levels of sodium or other minerals.
• The dish is easy to prepare and can be a complete, balanced meal.

33. Spinach and ricotta stuffed shells (low•fat ricotta)

Ingredient:

- 12 jumbo pasta shells
- 1 cup low•fat ricotta cheese
- 1 cup frozen chopped spinach, thawed and squeezed dry
- 1 egg, lightly beaten
- 2 tbsp grated Parmesan cheese
- 1 tsp dried oregano
- 1/4 tsp garlic powder
- 1/4 tsp black pepper
- 1 (24 oz) can low•sodium marinara sauce

Instructions:

1. Preheat oven to 375°F. Cook the pasta shells according to package instructions until al dente. Drain and set aside.

2. In a medium bowl, mix together the low•fat ricotta cheese, thawed and drained spinach, beaten egg, Parmesan cheese, oregano, garlic powder, and black pepper until well combined.

3. Spread 1/2 cup of the low•sodium marinara sauce in the bottom of a 9x13 inch baking dish.

4. Stuff each cooked pasta shell with a few tablespoons of the ricotta•spinach mixture and place in the baking dish.

5. Pour the remaining marinara sauce over the stuffed shells.

6. Cover the dish with foil and bake for 25•30 minutes, until heated through. Serve hot.

This dish is a great option for a renal diet as it uses low•fat ricotta cheese and low•sodium marinara sauce. The spinach provides vitamins and minerals, while the pasta shells offer complex carbohydrates. It's a flavorful and satisfying meal for seniors.

34. Spaghetti squash with garlic and herbs

Ingredient:

• 1 medium spaghetti squash, halved lengthwise and seeded
• 2 tbsp olive oil
• 3 cloves garlic, minced
• 2 tbsp chopped fresh parsley
• 1 tbsp chopped fresh basil
• 1/4 tsp black pepper
• Salt to taste (optional)

Instructions:

1. Preheat the oven to 400°F. Place the spaghetti squash halves cut·side down on a baking sheet. Bake for 40·50 minutes, until the squash is tender when pierced with a fork.

2. Remove the squash from the oven and let cool slightly. Use a fork to scrape the flesh into strands, transferring the "spaghetti" to a bowl.

3. In a small skillet, heat the olive oil over medium heat. Add the minced garlic and sauté for 1·2 minutes until fragrant.

4. Pour the garlic·infused oil over the spaghetti squash strands. Add the chopped parsley, basil, and black pepper. Toss everything together until well combined.

5. Taste and add a small amount of salt if desired, though the dish is flavorful without added salt.

6. Serve the spaghetti squash warm, as a main dish or side.

This spaghetti squash dish is an excellent low·carb, low·sodium option for a renal diet. The squash provides fiber, vitamins, and minerals, while the garlic, herbs, and olive oil add flavor without excess sodium. It's a simple, nutritious, and delicious meal for seniors.

35. Pesto pasta with pine nuts (low•sodium pesto)

Ingredient:

- 8 oz whole wheat pasta
- 1/2 cup low•sodium pesto (see recipe below)
- 2 tbsp toasted pine nuts

For the Low•Sodium Pesto:
- 2 cups fresh basil leaves
- 2 cloves garlic
- 2 tbsp pine nuts
- 2 tbsp olive oil
- 1 tbsp lemon juice
- 1/4 tsp salt

Instructions:

1. Bring a large pot of water to a boil. Cook the whole wheat pasta according to the package instructions until al dente. Drain the pasta and set it aside.

2. In a food processor or blender, combine all the ingredients for the low•sodium pesto: fresh basil leaves, garlic, pine nuts, olive oil, lemon juice, and salt. Blend until a smooth pesto forms.

3. In a large bowl, toss the cooked whole wheat pasta with the low•sodium pesto until the pasta is evenly coated.

4. Sprinkle the toasted pine nuts over the pesto pasta. Serve the pesto pasta with pine nuts warm.

This pesto pasta with pine nuts is a great option to support a renal diet for seniors over 60 for a few reasons:

- Whole wheat pasta is lower in phosphorus compared to regular pasta.
- The low•sodium pesto is made with fresh basil, garlic, pine nuts, olive oil, and a small amount of salt, keeping the sodium content down.
- Pine nuts provide a crunchy texture and additional nutrients without contributing high levels of potassium or phosphorus.
- The dish is easy to prepare and can be a flavorful, kidney•friendly meal.

You can also try adding some steamed or sautéed low•potassium vegetables, such as broccoli or zucchini, to the pesto pasta for extra nutrition.

36. Pork tenderloin with applesauce

Ingredient:

- 1 lb pork tenderloin
- 1 tsp dried thyme
- 1/2 tsp garlic powder
- 1/4 tsp black pepper
- 1 cup unsweetened applesauce
- 2 tbsp apple cider vinegar
- 1 tsp Dijon mustard
- Salt to taste (optional)

Instructions:

1. Preheat oven to 400°F. Line a baking sheet with foil or parchment paper.

2. In a small bowl, mix together the dried thyme, garlic powder, and black pepper. Rub this seasoning mixture all over the pork tenderloin.

3. Place the seasoned pork tenderloin on the prepared baking sheet. Roast for 20·25 minutes, until the internal temperature reaches 145°F.

4. While the pork is roasting, in a small saucepan, combine the unsweetened applesauce, apple cider vinegar, and Dijon mustard. Heat over medium, stirring occasionally, until warmed through.

5. Remove the pork tenderloin from the oven and let rest for 5 minutes before slicing.

6. Serve the sliced pork tenderloin with the warm applesauce on the side. Season with a small amount of salt if desired, but keep the sodium low.

This pork tenderloin dish is an excellent option for a renal diet. Pork is a lean protein, and the unsweetened applesauce provides natural sweetness without added sugars. The simple seasoning keeps the sodium content low. It's a flavorful and nutritious meal for seniors.

37. Lemon herb chicken breasts

Ingredient:

- 4 boneless, skinless chicken breasts
- 2 tbsp olive oil
- 2 tbsp fresh lemon juice
- 1 tsp dried oregano
- 1 tsp dried basil
- 1/2 tsp garlic powder
- 1/4 tsp black pepper
- Salt to taste (optional)
- Lemon wedges for serving

Instructions:

1. Preheat oven to 400°F. Line a baking sheet with parchment paper or foil.

2. In a shallow dish, combine the olive oil, lemon juice, oregano, basil, garlic powder, and black pepper. Add the chicken breasts and turn to coat them evenly in the marinade.

3. Arrange the marinated chicken breasts on the prepared baking sheet.

4. Bake for 25·30 minutes, until the chicken is cooked through and reaches an internal temperature of 165°F.

5. Remove the chicken from the oven and let it rest for 5 minutes.

6. Serve the lemon herb chicken breasts warm, with a small amount of salt added if desired, though the dish should be low in sodium. Garnish with lemon wedges.

This lemon herb chicken is an excellent choice for a renal diet. Chicken is a lean protein, and the lemon, herbs, and spices add flavor without the need for excess sodium. The simple preparation makes it an easy, healthy meal for seniors. Pair it with roasted vegetables or a side salad for a complete, kidney·friendly dinner.

38. Beef kebabs with bell peppers and onions

Ingredient:

- 1 lb lean beef sirloin, cut into 1·inch cubes
- 1 red bell pepper, cut into 1·inch pieces
- 1 green bell pepper, cut into 1·inch pieces
- 1 red onion, cut into 1·inch pieces
- 2 tbsp olive oil
- 1 tsp dried oregano
- 1/2 tsp garlic powder
- 1/4 tsp black pepper
- Salt to taste (optional)
- Lemon wedges for serving (optional)

Instructions:

1. Preheat grill or grill pan to medium·high heat.

2. In a large bowl, toss the beef cubes, bell pepper pieces, and onion pieces with the olive oil, oregano, garlic powder, and black pepper until well coated.

3. Thread the beef and vegetables onto metal or wooden skewers, leaving a small space between each item.

4. Grill the kebabs for 12·15 minutes, turning occasionally, until the beef is cooked through and the vegetables are tender.

5. Season with a small amount of salt if desired, though the dish should be low in sodium.

6. Serve the beef kebabs hot, with lemon wedges on the side if desired.

This beef kebab dish is a great option for a renal diet. The lean beef provides protein, while the bell peppers and onions add fiber, vitamins, and minerals. By avoiding added salt and using just a few herbs and spices for seasoning, the sodium content is kept low. It's a flavorful and nutritious meal for seniors.

39. Turkey chili (low•sodium)

Ingredient:

- 1 lb ground turkey
- 1 onion, diced
- 3 cloves garlic, minced
- 1 (15 oz) can no•salt•added diced tomatoes
- 1 (15 oz) can no•salt•added kidney beans, rinsed and drained
- 1 (15 oz) can no•salt•added black beans, rinsed and drained
- 2 cups low•sodium chicken or vegetable broth
- 2 tbsp chili powder
- 1 tsp ground cumin
- 1 tsp dried oregano
- 1/4 tsp cayenne pepper (optional)
- 1/4 tsp black pepper
- Salt to taste (optional)

Instructions:

1. In a large pot or Dutch oven, cook the ground turkey over medium heat until browned and crumbled, 5•7 minutes. Drain any excess fat.

2. Add the diced onion and minced garlic to the pot. Sauté for 2•3 minutes until the onion is translucent.

3. Stir in the no•salt•added diced tomatoes, kidney beans, black beans, and low•sodium broth.

4. Add the chili powder, cumin, oregano, cayenne (if using), and black pepper. Stir to combine.

5. Bring the chili to a simmer and let it cook for 20•25 minutes, stirring occasionally, until thickened.

6. Taste and add a small amount of salt if needed, but keep the sodium content low.

7. Serve the low•sodium turkey chili hot, garnished with chopped fresh herbs or scallions if desired.

This turkey chili is an excellent option for a renal diet. The lean ground turkey provides protein, while the beans offer fiber and additional protein. By using no•salt•added canned goods and limiting added salt, the sodium content is kept low. It's a hearty and nutritious meal for seniors.

40. Stuffed bell peppers with ground turkey and quinoa

Ingredient:

- 4 medium bell peppers, halved lengthwise and seeded
- 1 lb ground turkey
- 1 cup cooked quinoa
- 1 cup diced onion
- 2 cloves garlic, minced
- 1 (14.5 oz) can no·salt·added diced tomatoes
- 2 tbsp chopped fresh parsley
- 1 tsp dried oregano
- 1/4 tsp black pepper
- Salt to taste (optional)

Instructions:

1. Preheat oven to 375°F. Place the bell pepper halves in a baking dish and set aside.

2. In a large skillet over medium heat, cook the ground turkey, onion, and garlic until the turkey is browned and the vegetables are tender, about 7·10 minutes. Drain any excess fat.

3. Stir in the cooked quinoa, no·salt·added diced tomatoes, parsley, oregano, and black pepper. Taste and add a small amount of salt if needed, but keep the sodium low.

4. Spoon the turkey·quinoa mixture evenly into the bell pepper halves.

5. Cover the baking dish with foil and bake for 30·35 minutes, until the peppers are tender.

6. Remove the foil and bake for an additional 5 minutes to lightly brown the tops.

7. Serve the stuffed bell peppers hot.

This dish is an excellent choice for a renal diet. The ground turkey provides protein, the quinoa offers complex carbs, and the bell peppers are packed with vitamins and fiber. By using no·salt·added canned tomatoes and limiting added salt, the sodium content is kept low. It's a nutritious and flavorful meal for seniors.

41. Lentil soup (low•sodium)

Ingredient:

- 1 cup dry brown or green lentils, rinsed
- 4 cups low•sodium vegetable or chicken broth
- 1 cup diced carrots
- 1 cup diced celery
- 1 cup diced onion
- 2 cloves garlic, minced
- 1 tsp dried thyme
- 1 bay leaf
- 1/4 tsp black pepper
- Salt to taste (optional)
- Chopped parsley for garnish (optional)

Instructions:

1. In a large pot, combine the rinsed lentils and low•sodium broth. Bring to a boil over high heat.

2. Reduce heat to medium•low, then add the diced carrots, celery, onion, and minced garlic. Simmer for 20•25 minutes, until the lentils and vegetables are tender.

3. Stir in the dried thyme and bay leaf. Season with a small amount of black pepper.

4. Taste and add a pinch of salt If needed, but keep in mind the soup should be low in sodium.

5. Ladle the lentil soup into bowls and garnish with chopped parsley if desired.

This lentil soup is an excellent source of plant•based protein, fiber, and complex carbohydrates, all of which are important for a renal diet. The low•sodium broth and lack of added salt make it kidney•friendly. It's a hearty, comforting, and nutritious meal for seniors.

42. Veggie stir·fry with tofu

Ingredient:

- 1 block (14 oz) extra·firm tofu, cubed
- 2 tbsp low·sodium soy sauce or tamari
- 1 tbsp rice vinegar
- 1 tsp sesame oil
- 1 tbsp olive oil
- 2 cups mixed vegetables (such as broccoli, bell peppers, snap peas, carrots)
- 1 cup sliced mushrooms
- 3 cloves garlic, minced
- 1 tsp grated fresh ginger
- 1/4 tsp red pepper flakes (optional)
- 2 cups cooked brown rice

Instructions:

1. In a small bowl, combine the cubed tofu, low·sodium soy sauce or tamari, rice vinegar, and sesame oil. Toss to coat the tofu and set aside.

2. Heat the olive oil in a large skillet or wok over medium·high heat. Add the mixed vegetables and mushrooms. Stir·fry for 5·7 minutes until the vegetables are tender·crisp.

3. Add the marinated tofu, garlic, ginger, and red pepper flakes (if using). Stir·fry for an additional 3·5 minutes until the tofu is heated through.

4. Serve the veggie and tofu stir·fry over the cooked brown rice.

This stir·fry is a great option for a renal diet. Tofu is a lean protein that is low in sodium, and the vegetables provide fiber, vitamins, and minerals. The low·sodium soy sauce or tamari keeps the sodium content in check. Brown rice offers complex carbohydrates. It's a balanced, flavorful, and kidney·friendly meal.

43. Chickpea curry with brown rice

Ingredient:

- 1 cup uncooked brown rice
- 1 tbsp olive oil
- 1 onion, diced
- 3 cloves garlic, minced
- 1 tbsp grated fresh ginger
- 2 tsp curry powder
- 1 tsp ground cumin
- 1/4 tsp cayenne pepper (optional)
- 1 (15 oz) can no·salt·added chickpeas, rinsed and drained
- 1 (14 oz) can no·salt·added diced tomatoes
- 1 cup low·sodium vegetable or chicken broth
- 1 cup frozen peas
- 1/4 cup chopped fresh cilantro (optional)
- Salt and pepper to taste

Instructions:

1. Cook the brown rice according to package instructions.

2. In a large skillet or saucepan, heat the olive oil over medium heat. Add the diced onion and sauté for 5 minutes until translucent.

3. Stir in the minced garlic and grated ginger. Cook for 1 minute until fragrant.

4. Add the curry powder, cumin, and cayenne (if using). Stir to coat the onions and cook for 2 minutes.

5. Pour in the no·salt·added chickpeas, diced tomatoes, and low·sodium broth. Bring to a simmer and cook for 10·15 minutes, until slightly thickened.

6. Stir in the frozen peas and cook for 2·3 minutes until heated through.

7. Remove from heat and stir in the chopped cilantro, if using. Season with a small amount of salt and pepper to taste. Serve the chickpea curry over the cooked brown rice.

This chickpea curry is a great option for a renal diet. Chickpeas are a good source of plant·based protein and fiber, while the brown rice provides complex carbohydrates. The low·sodium broth and canned goods keep the sodium content in check. It's a flavorful, nutritious, and kidney·friendly meal.

44. Quinoa stuffed peppers

Ingredient:

- 4 medium bell peppers, halved lengthwise and seeded
- 1 cup cooked quinoa
- 1 (15 oz) can no•salt•added diced tomatoes
- 1 cup cooked black beans, rinsed and drained
- 1/2 cup crumbled feta cheese (optional)
- 2 tbsp chopped fresh parsley
- 1 tsp dried oregano
- 1/4 tsp garlic powder
- 1/4 tsp black pepper
- Salt to taste (optional)

Instructions:

1. Preheat oven to 375°F. Place the bell pepper halves in a baking dish and set aside.

2. In a medium bowl, combine the cooked quinoa, no•salt•added diced tomatoes, black beans, crumbled feta (if using), parsley, oregano, garlic powder, and black pepper. Stir to mix well.

3. Spoon the quinoa mixture evenly into the bell pepper halves, packing it in gently.

4. Cover the baking dish with foil and bake for 30•35 minutes, until the peppers are tender.

5. Remove the foil and bake for an additional 5 minutes to lightly brown the tops.

6. Serve the quinoa stuffed peppers hot. Add a small amount of salt if desired, but keep the sodium content low.

These quinoa stuffed peppers are an excellent choice for a renal diet. Quinoa is a high•protein, high•fiber grain, and the black beans provide additional plant•based protein. The bell peppers are packed with vitamins and minerals. By using no•salt•added canned goods and limiting added salt, this dish is kidney•friendly. It's a nutritious and flavorful meal for seniors.

45. Black bean burgers on whole wheat buns

Ingredient:

- 1 (15 oz) can no•salt•added black beans, rinsed and drained
- 1/2 cup cooked quinoa
- 1/4 cup whole wheat breadcrumbs
- 1 egg, lightly beaten
- 1 tbsp olive oil
- 1 tsp chili powder
- 1/2 tsp ground cumin
- 1/4 tsp garlic powder
- 1/4 tsp black pepper
- 4 whole wheat hamburger buns
- Toppings (such as lettuce, tomato, onion)

Instructions:

1. In a medium bowl, mash the rinsed and drained black beans with a fork or potato masher.

2. Stir in the cooked quinoa, whole wheat breadcrumbs, beaten egg, olive oil, chili powder, cumin, garlic powder, and black pepper until well combined.

3. Divide the black bean mixture into 4 equal portions and shape them into patties, about 4 inches wide and 1/2 inch thick.

4. Heat a large skillet or grill pan over medium heat. Cook the black bean patties for 4•5 minutes per side, until lightly browned and heated through.

5. Serve the black bean burgers on the whole wheat buns, topped with your desired toppings.

These black bean burgers are a great option for a renal diet. Black beans are a good source of plant•based protein and fiber, while the whole wheat buns provide complex carbohydrates. The simple seasoning keeps the sodium content low. It's a nutritious and satisfying meal for seniors.

46. Grilled shrimp skewers

Ingredient:

• 1 lb large shrimp, peeled and deveined
• 2 tbsp olive oil
• 1 tbsp lemon juice
• 1 tsp dried oregano
• 1/2 tsp garlic powder
• 1/4 tsp black pepper
• Salt to taste (optional)
• Lemon wedges for serving

Instructions:

1. In a medium bowl, combine the shrimp, olive oil, lemon juice, oregano, garlic powder, and black pepper. Toss to coat the shrimp evenly.

2. Thread the shrimp onto metal or wooden skewers, leaving a small space between each shrimp.

3. Preheat grill or grill pan to medium•high heat.

4. Grill the shrimp skewers for 2•3 minutes per side, until the shrimp are opaque and cooked through.

5. Season with a small amount of salt if desired, though the dish should be low in sodium.

6. Serve the grilled shrimp skewers hot, with lemon wedges on the side.

This grilled shrimp dish is an excellent option for a renal diet. Shrimp is a lean protein that is low in sodium. The simple seasoning of lemon, herbs, and spices adds flavor without excess sodium. Grilling the shrimp keeps the preparation light and healthy. Serve this as a main dish or appetizer for seniors on a renal diet.

47. Seared scallops with citrus glaze

Ingredient:

- 1 lb sea scallops, patted dry
- 1 tbsp olive oil
- 2 tbsp freshly squeezed orange juice
- 1 tbsp freshly squeezed lemon juice
- 1 tsp honey
- 1/4 tsp grated orange zest
- 1/4 tsp black pepper
- Salt to taste (optional)
- Chopped parsley for garnish (optional)

Instructions:

1. In a small bowl, whisk together the orange juice, lemon juice, honey, and orange zest to make the citrus glaze. Set aside.

2. Heat the olive oil in a large skillet over medium•high heat.

3. Pat the scallops dry with paper towels and season lightly with a small amount of salt, if desired.

4. Sear the scallops in the hot skillet for 2•3 minutes per side, until they develop a golden•brown crust and are opaque in the center.

5. Reduce the heat to low and pour the citrus glaze into the skillet. Gently toss the scallops to coat them in the glaze.

6. Cook for an additional 1•2 minutes, until the glaze has thickened slightly.

7. Remove the seared scallops with the citrus glaze from the heat.

8. Serve the scallops immediately, garnished with chopped parsley if desired.

This seared scallop dish is an excellent choice for a renal diet. Scallops are a lean, low•sodium protein. The citrus glaze adds flavor without excessive sodium. It's a simple yet elegant meal that is both delicious and kidney•friendly for seniors.

48. Baked cod with tomatoes and olives

Ingredient:

- 1 lb cod fillets
- 1 (14.5 oz) can no•salt•added diced tomatoes
- 1/4 cup pitted and sliced black olives
- 2 tbsp olive oil
- 1 tsp dried oregano
- 1/2 tsp garlic powder
- 1/4 tsp black pepper
- Salt to taste (optional)
- Chopped parsley for garnish (optional)

Instructions:

1. Preheat the oven to 400°F. Lightly grease a baking dish with a small amount of olive oil.

2. Place the cod fillets in the prepared baking dish.

3. In a medium bowl, combine the no•salt•added diced tomatoes, sliced black olives, olive oil, dried oregano, garlic powder, and black pepper. Stir to mix well.

4. Spoon the tomato•olive mixture over the top of the cod fillets, making sure to distribute it evenly.

5. Bake for 18•22 minutes, until the cod is opaque and flakes easily with a fork.

6. Remove the baked cod from the oven and season with a small amount of salt if desired, but keep the sodium content low.

7. Garnish with chopped parsley, if desired.

8. Serve the baked cod with tomatoes and olives immediately.

This baked cod dish is an excellent choice for a renal diet. Cod is a lean, low•sodium fish, and the tomatoes and olives provide flavor without excess sodium. It's a simple, one•pan meal that is both nutritious and delicious for seniors.

49. Shrimp and vegetable stir·fry

Ingredient:

- 1 lb shrimp, peeled and deveined
- 2 tbsp low·sodium soy sauce or tamari
- 1 tbsp rice vinegar
- 1 tsp sesame oil
- 1 tbsp olive oil
- 2 cups mixed vegetables (such as broccoli, snap peas, bell peppers, carrots)
- 3 cloves garlic, minced
- 1 tsp grated fresh ginger
- 1/4 tsp red pepper flakes (optional)
- 2 cups cooked brown rice

Instructions:

1. In a small bowl, combine the shrimp, low·sodium soy sauce or tamari, rice vinegar, and sesame oil. Toss to coat the shrimp and set aside.

2. Heat the olive oil in a large skillet or wok over medium·high heat. Add the mixed vegetables and stir·fry for 5·7 minutes until tender·crisp.

3. Add the marinated shrimp, minced garlic, grated ginger, and red pepper flakes (if using). Stir·fry for an additional 3·5 minutes until the shrimp are opaque and cooked through.

4. Serve the shrimp and vegetable stir·fry over the cooked brown rice.

This shrimp and vegetable stir·fry is a great option for a renal diet. Shrimp is a lean protein that is low in sodium, and the vegetables provide fiber, vitamins, and minerals. The low·sodium soy sauce or tamari keeps the sodium content in check. Brown rice offers complex carbohydrates. It's a balanced, flavorful, and kidney·friendly meal.

50. Crab cakes with low•sodium remoulade

Ingredient:

- 1 lb lump crabmeat, picked over for shells
- 1/2 cup panko breadcrumbs
- 2 tablespoons mayonnaise
- 1 egg, lightly beaten
- 2 tablespoons chopped fresh parsley
- 1 tablespoon Dijon mustard
- 1 teaspoon lemon zest
- 1/4 teaspoon cayenne pepper
- Salt and pepper to taste

Low•Sodium Remoulade Sauce:

- 1/2 cup low•fat mayonnaise
- 2 tablespoons Dijon mustard
- 1 tablespoon lemon juice
- 1 tablespoon chopped fresh parsley
- 1 teaspoon capers, rinsed and chopped
- 1/4 teaspoon paprika
- 1/8 teaspoon cayenne pepper
- Salt and pepper to taste

Instructions:

1. For the crab cakes, gently mix together all the crab cake ingredients in a bowl until just combined. Form the mixture into 8 equal•sized patties, about 1/2 inch thick.

2. Heat a large nonstick skillet over medium heat and add enough oil to lightly coat the bottom. Working in batches if needed, cook the crab cakes for 3•4 minutes per side until golden brown.

3. For the remoulade sauce, whisk together all the sauce ingredients in a small bowl. Season with salt and pepper to taste.

4. Serve the warm crab cakes with the low•sodium remoulade sauce on the side for dipping. Enjoy!

The key to the low•sodium remoulade is using low•fat mayonnaise and limiting the amount of added salt. This makes it a healthier accompaniment to the crab cakes.

51. Baked apples with cinnamon

Ingredient:

- 4 medium·sized apples (such as Gala, Honeycrisp, or Fuji)
- 1/4 cup brown sugar
- 1 teaspoon ground cinnamon
- 1/4 teaspoon ground nutmeg
- 2 tablespoons unsalted butter, softened
- 1/4 cup old·fashioned oats
- 2 tablespoons chopped walnuts or pecans (optional)
- Vanilla ice cream or whipped cream for serving (optional)

Instructions:

1. Preheat your oven to 375°F (190°C).

2. Wash and core the apples, leaving about 1/2 inch of the core at the bottom to hold the filling. Place the apples in a baking dish.

3. In a small bowl, mix together the brown sugar, cinnamon, and nutmeg. Spoon this mixture evenly into the center of each apple.

4. In another small bowl, combine the softened butter, oats, and chopped nuts (if using). Spoon this mixture over the top of the filled apples.

5. Pour about 1/4 cup of water into the bottom of the baking dish to prevent the apples from burning.

6. Bake the apples for 30·40 minutes, or until they are tender when pierced with a fork. The apples should be slightly caramelized on top.

7. Serve the baked apples warm, with a scoop of vanilla ice cream or a dollop of whipped cream, if desired.

Enjoy this simple and delicious baked apple dessert! The cinnamon and nutmeg flavors pair perfectly with the sweet, tender apples.

52. Low·fat yogurt parfait with granola and berries

Ingredient:

• 2 cups low·fat or non·fat plain Greek yogurt
• 1 cup fresh berries (such as blueberries, raspberries, or sliced strawberries)
• 1 cup low·fat granola

Instructions:

1. In a parfait glass or small bowl, layer the ingredients as follows:
    • 1/4 cup yogurt
    • 1/4 cup granola
    • 1/4 cup berries
    • Repeat the layers two more times, ending with the berries on top.

2. Repeat the layering process with the remaining yogurt, granola, and berries to make 4 parfaits total.

3. Refrigerate the parfaits until ready to serve, at least 30 minutes.

Tips:
• Use a variety of berries for a colorful and flavorful parfait.

• Choose a low·fat or non·fat granola that is low in added sugars.

• You can also use plain low·fat or non·fat regular yogurt instead of Greek yogurt.

• For extra crunch, sprinkle a few chopped nuts or toasted coconut on top.

• Drizzle a small amount of honey or maple syrup over the layers if you want a sweeter parfait.

This low·fat yogurt parfait is a healthy and delicious breakfast or snack option. The combination of creamy yogurt, crunchy granola, and fresh berries makes for a satisfying and nutritious treat.

53. Angel food cake with strawberries

Ingredient:

• 1 angel food cake, store•bought or homemade
• 2 cups fresh strawberries, sliced
• 1 tbsp honey (optional)

Instructions:

1. Prepare the angel food cake according to package or recipe instructions. Allow the cake to cool completely.

2. In a medium bowl, gently toss the sliced fresh strawberries. If desired, drizzle with a small amount of honey to lightly sweeten the berries.

3. Slice the angel food cake and serve each portion topped with the fresh strawberries.

This dessert is a great option for a renal diet. Angel food cake is low in fat and sodium, and the fresh strawberries provide natural sweetness without added sugars. The honey is optional, as the strawberries are already quite sweet on their own.

Angel food cake is a light and airy dessert that is easy to digest. The combination of the fluffy cake and juicy, flavorful strawberries makes for a refreshing and satisfying treat. This dessert is a good source of carbohydrates and provides a touch of natural sweetness, all while being kidney•friendly.

54. Rice pudding (made with low•fat milk)

Ingredient:

- 1/2 cup uncooked short•grain white rice
- 2 cups low•fat milk
- 1/4 cup white sugar
- 1 tsp vanilla extract
- 1/4 tsp ground cinnamon
- 1/8 tsp ground nutmeg

Instructions:

1. In a medium saucepan, combine the uncooked rice and low•fat milk. Bring to a gentle simmer over medium heat, stirring frequently.

2. Once the mixture begins to simmer, reduce heat to low and continue cooking, stirring occasionally, for 25•30 minutes, until the rice is tender and the pudding has thickened.

3. Stir in the white sugar and vanilla extract. Cook for an additional 5 minutes, continuing to stir.

4. Remove the rice pudding from heat and stir in the ground cinnamon and nutmeg.

5. Serve the rice pudding warm or chilled. If desired, top with an extra sprinkle of cinnamon.

55. Sorbet (low•potassium flavors)

Ingredient:

- 2 cups water
- 1 cup white sugar
- 1/2 cup lemon juice
- 1/2 tsp lemon zest
- 1/4 tsp vanilla extract

Instructions:

1. In a small saucepan, combine the water and sugar. Bring to a boil over medium heat, stirring occasionally until the sugar has dissolved. Remove from heat and let cool completely.

2. Once the sugar syrup has cooled, stir in the lemon juice, lemon zest, and vanilla extract.

3. Pour the lemon sorbet mixture into a shallow baking dish or metal pan. Place in the freezer and stir every 30 minutes for the first 2 hours, then every hour thereafter, until completely frozen, about 4•6 hours total.

4. Once fully frozen, scoop the lemon sorbet into individual servings.

This lemon sorbet is a great low•potassium dessert option for a renal diet. Lemon is a low•potassium fruit, and the small amount of sugar and lack of dairy ingredients make it kidney•friendly. The sorbet provides a refreshing, icy treat without the high potassium content of many other fruit•based desserts. It's a light and flavorful way for seniors to enjoy a sweet treat while adhering to a renal diet.

Other low•potassium sorbet flavor ideas include:
- Lime
- Raspberry
- Mango
- Pineapple

56. Spinach salad with strawberries and balsamic vinaigrette

Ingredient:

- 5 oz baby spinach
- 1 cup fresh strawberries, sliced
- 2 tbsp crumbled feta cheese (optional)
- 2 tbsp balsamic vinegar
- 1 tbsp olive oil
- 1 tsp Dijon mustard
- 1 tsp honey
- 1/4 tsp black pepper
- Salt to taste (optional)

Instructions:

1. In a large salad bowl, combine the baby spinach, sliced strawberries, and crumbled feta cheese (if using).

2. In a small bowl, whisk together the balsamic vinegar, olive oil, Dijon mustard, honey, and black pepper to make the vinaigrette dressing.

3. Drizzle the balsamic vinaigrette over the spinach salad and toss gently to coat.

4. Taste the salad and add a small amount of salt if desired, but keep the sodium content low.

5. Serve the spinach salad with strawberries immediately.

This spinach salad is an excellent choice for a renal diet. Spinach is packed with vitamins, minerals, and antioxidants, while the fresh strawberries provide natural sweetness. The balsamic vinaigrette is low in sodium, allowing the flavors of the produce to shine. The optional feta cheese adds a creamy, tangy element. It's a refreshing and nutritious salad for seniors.

57. Greek salad with feta cheese and olives (low·sodium dressing)

Ingredient:

- 6 cups chopped romaine lettuce
- 1 cup diced cucumber
- 1/2 cup diced tomatoes
- 1/4 cup crumbled low·fat feta cheese
- 2 tbsp sliced black olives
- 2 tbsp olive oil
- 1 tbsp red wine vinegar
- 1 tsp dried oregano
- 1/4 tsp garlic powder
- 1/8 tsp black pepper
- Salt to taste (optional)

Instructions:

1. In a large salad bowl, combine the chopped romaine lettuce, diced cucumber, diced tomatoes, crumbled low·fat feta cheese, and sliced black olives.

2. In a small bowl, whisk together the olive oil, red wine vinegar, dried oregano, garlic powder, and black pepper to make the dressing.

3. Drizzle the low·sodium dressing over the salad and toss gently to coat.

4. Taste the salad and add a small amount of salt if desired, but keep the sodium content low.

5. Serve the Greek salad immediately.

This Greek salad is an excellent choice for a renal diet. The vegetables provide fiber, vitamins, and minerals, while the feta cheese and olives add flavor without excessive sodium. The simple olive oil and vinegar dressing keeps the sodium low. It's a refreshing and nutritious salad for seniors.

58. Waldorf salad with low•fat mayonnaise

Ingredient:

- 2 apples, diced
- 1 cup diced celery
- 1/2 cup halved grapes
- 1/4 cup chopped walnuts
- 2 tbsp low•fat mayonnaise
- 1 tbsp lemon juice
- 1 tsp honey
- 1/4 tsp ground cinnamon
- Black pepper to taste
- Salt to taste (optional)

Instructions:

1. In a large bowl, combine the diced apples, diced celery, halved grapes, and chopped walnuts.

2. In a small bowl, whisk together the low•fat mayonnaise, lemon juice, honey, and ground cinnamon to make the dressing.

3. Pour the dressing over the fruit and vegetable mixture and toss gently to coat.

4. Season with a small amount of black pepper and salt, if desired, but keep the sodium content low.

5. Refrigerate the Waldorf salad for at least 30 minutes to allow the flavors to meld.

6. Serve chilled.

This Waldorf salad is a great option for a renal diet. The apples, celery, and grapes provide fiber, vitamins, and natural sweetness. The walnuts add a crunchy texture and healthy fats. By using low•fat mayonnaise, the saturated fat and sodium content are reduced. It's a refreshing and nutritious salad for seniors.

59. Quinoa tabbouleh with cucumber and mint

Ingredient:

• 1 cup cooked quinoa, cooled
• 1 cup diced cucumber
• 1/2 cup chopped fresh parsley
• 1/4 cup chopped fresh mint
• 2 tbsp lemon juice
• 1 tbsp olive oil
• 1/4 tsp ground cumin
• 1/4 tsp black pepper
• Salt to taste (optional)

Instructions:

1. In a large bowl, combine the cooked and cooled quinoa, diced cucumber, chopped parsley, and chopped mint.

2. In a small bowl, whisk together the lemon juice, olive oil, ground cumin, and black pepper to make the dressing.

3. Pour the dressing over the quinoa and vegetable mixture and toss gently to coat.

4. Taste the tabbouleh and add a small amount of salt if desired, but keep the sodium content low.

5. Cover and refrigerate the quinoa tabbouleh for at least 30 minutes to allow the flavors to meld.

6. Serve chilled or at room temperature.

This quinoa tabbouleh salad is an excellent choice for a renal diet. Quinoa is a high•protein, high•fiber grain that is low in sodium. The fresh cucumber, parsley, and mint provide vitamins, minerals, and antioxidants. The simple lemon and olive oil dressing keeps the sodium content in check. It's a refreshing, flavorful, and nutritious salad for seniors.

60. Bean salad with kidney beans and vinaigrette dressing

Ingredient:

- 1 (15 oz) can no·salt·added kidney beans, rinsed and drained
- 1 (15 oz) can no·salt·added garbanzo beans, rinsed and drained
- 1 cup diced celery
- 1/2 cup diced red onion
- 1/4 cup chopped fresh parsley
- 2 tbsp olive oil
- 2 tbsp red wine vinegar
- 1 tsp Dijon mustard
- 1 tsp dried oregano
- 1/4 tsp black pepper
- Salt to taste (optional)

Instructions:

1. In a large bowl, combine the no·salt·added kidney beans, garbanzo beans, diced celery, diced red onion, and chopped parsley. Toss to mix.

2. In a small bowl, whisk together the olive oil, red wine vinegar, Dijon mustard, dried oregano, and black pepper to make the vinaigrette dressing.

3. Pour the vinaigrette dressing over the bean salad and toss gently to coat.

4. Taste the salad and add a small amount of salt if desired, but keep the sodium content low.

5. Cover and refrigerate the bean salad for at least 30 minutes to allow the flavors to meld.

6. Serve chilled or at room temperature.

This bean salad is a great option for a renal diet. The combination of kidney beans and garbanzo beans provides plant·based protein and fiber. The simple vinaigrette dressing is low in sodium, allowing the natural flavors of the vegetables to shine. It's a refreshing and nutritious side dish or light main course for seniors.

61. Turkey and avocado wrap

Ingredient:

- 4 whole wheat tortillas or wraps
- 8 oz sliced turkey breast
- 1 avocado, sliced
- 1 cup shredded lettuce
- 2 tablespoons low·fat mayonnaise or Greek yogurt
- 1 tablespoon Dijon mustard
- Salt and pepper to taste

Instructions:

1. In a small bowl, mix together the mayonnaise (or Greek yogurt) and Dijon mustard. Season with a pinch of salt and pepper.

2. Lay the tortillas or wraps out on a clean surface. Spread the mayonnaise/mustard mixture evenly over each wrap.

3. Divide the turkey slices evenly among the wraps, placing them in the center.

4. Top the turkey with sliced avocado and shredded lettuce.

5. Fold the bottom of the wrap up over the filling, then fold in the sides and continue rolling tightly into a wrap.

6. Slice the wraps in half diagonally, if desired, and serve.

Tips:
- Use a whole wheat or spinach tortilla/wrap for added fiber and nutrients.
- You can also add other veggies like tomato, onion, or sprouts.
- For extra flavor, try adding a sprinkle of shredded cheese or a drizzle of balsamic glaze.
- Wrap tightly in foil or parchment paper to pack for lunch or on·the·go.

This turkey and avocado wrap is a healthy, satisfying, and portable meal or snack. The creamy avocado, lean turkey, and crunchy lettuce make for a delicious flavor and texture combination.

62. Grilled vegetable panini
with low·sodium cheese

Ingredient:

- 4 whole wheat tortillas or wraps
- 8 oz sliced turkey breast
- 1 avocado, sliced
- 1/2 cup shredded lettuce
- 2 tbsp low·fat plain Greek yogurt
- 1 tbsp lemon juice
- 1/4 tsp garlic powder
- Black pepper to taste
- Salt to taste (optional)

Instructions:

1. In a small bowl, mix together the low·fat plain Greek yogurt, lemon juice, and garlic powder to make a creamy dressing.

2. Lay the whole wheat tortillas or wraps on a flat surface. Evenly distribute the sliced turkey, avocado slices, and shredded lettuce onto the center of each wrap.

3. Drizzle the yogurt·lemon dressing over the fillings.

4. Season with black pepper and a small amount of salt if desired, but keep the sodium content low.

5. Fold the bottom of the wrap up over the fillings, then fold in the sides and continue rolling tightly into a wrap.

6. Serve the turkey and avocado wraps immediately.

This turkey and avocado wrap is a great option for a renal diet. Turkey is a lean protein, and avocado provides healthy fats and fiber. The low·fat Greek yogurt dressing adds creaminess without excess sodium or saturated fat. The whole wheat wrap offers complex carbohydrates. It's a balanced and nutritious meal or snack for seniors.

63. Egg salad on whole wheat bread

Ingredient:

- 6 hard•boiled eggs, peeled and chopped
- 2 tbsp low•fat mayonnaise
- 1 tsp Dijon mustard
- 1 tbsp chopped fresh parsley
- 1/4 tsp black pepper
- Salt to taste (optional)
- 8 slices whole wheat bread

Instructions:

1. In a medium bowl, combine the chopped hard•boiled eggs, low•fat mayonnaise, Dijon mustard, chopped parsley, and black pepper. Stir gently until well mixed.

2. Taste the egg salad and add a small amount of salt if desired, but keep the sodium content low.

3. Divide the egg salad evenly between 4 slices of whole wheat bread. Top with the remaining 4 slices of bread to make 4 egg salad sandwiches.

4. Serve the egg salad sandwiches immediately, or refrigerate until ready to serve.

This egg salad on whole wheat bread is a great option for a renal diet. Eggs are a high•quality protein source, and the whole wheat bread provides complex carbohydrates. The low•fat mayonnaise and limited added salt help keep the sodium content in check. It's a simple, nutritious, and satisfying meal or snack for seniors.

64. Chicken salad on whole grain pita

Ingredient:

• 2 cups cooked, diced chicken breast
• 1/4 cup low•fat plain Greek yogurt
• 1 tablespoon Dijon mustard
• 1 tablespoon lemon juice
• 1/4 cup diced celery
• 2 tablespoons diced onion
• 1/4 cup diced apple
• 2 tablespoons chopped parsley
• Salt and pepper to taste
• 4 whole grain pita pockets, halved

Instructions:

1. In a medium bowl, combine the diced chicken, Greek yogurt, Dijon mustard, and lemon juice. Mix well until the chicken is evenly coated.

2. Fold in the diced celery, onion, apple, and chopped parsley. Season with a pinch of salt and pepper. Scoop the chicken salad mixture into the halved whole grain pita pockets.

Nutritional Considerations for a Renal Diet:

• Chicken is a lean protein source, which is important for seniors with kidney disease.

• Greek yogurt provides protein and calcium without the high sodium content of regular mayonnaise.

• Whole grain pita is a good source of complex carbohydrates and fiber, which can help manage blood sugar levels.

• Celery, onion, and apple add flavor and texture without contributing excessive potassium or phosphorus.

• Lemon juice and parsley are low in sodium, potassium, and phosphorus, making them kidney•friendly.

This chicken salad on whole grain pita is a nutritious and flavorful option for seniors following a renal diet. The combination of lean protein, complex carbs, and fresh vegetables makes it a balanced and satisfying meal.

65. Hummus and vegetable sandwich

Ingredient:

- 4 slices whole grain or multigrain bread
- 1/2 cup hummus (your favorite flavor)
- 1 cup mixed vegetables, thinly sliced (such as cucumber, tomato, bell pepper, carrots, sprouts)
- 2 ounces crumbled feta cheese (optional)
- Salt and pepper to taste

Instructions:

1. Toast the bread slices until lightly golden brown.

2. Spread about 2•3 tablespoons of hummus evenly over each slice of toast.

3. Layer the sliced vegetables over the hummus on two of the bread slices.

4. If using, sprinkle the crumbled feta cheese over the vegetables.

5. Season with a pinch of salt and pepper.

6. Top the vegetable•topped slices with the remaining two slices of toast to create a sandwich.

7. Cut the sandwiches in half diagonally, if desired.

Variations:
- Use different types of hummus flavors like roasted red pepper, garlic, or sun•dried tomato.

- Add other toppings like avocado slices, sprouts, or a drizzle of balsamic glaze.

- Use a variety of vegetables like zucchini, eggplant, or radish for different textures and flavors. For a heartier sandwich, add a slice of cheese or a few slices of turkey or roast beef.

This hummus and vegetable sandwich is a delicious, nutritious, and satisfying meatless option. The creamy hummus paired with the crunchy, fresh veggies makes for a flavorful and filling lunch or snack.

66. Vegetable Frittata with low·fat cheese

Ingredient:

• 8 large eggs
• 1/4 cup low·fat milk
• 1/4 tsp black pepper
• 1 tbsp olive oil
• 1 cup diced bell peppers
• 1 cup diced zucchini
• 1/2 cup diced onion
• 2 cloves garlic, minced
• 1/2 cup shredded low·fat cheddar or mozzarella cheese

Instructions:

1. Preheat oven to 375°F.

2. In a medium bowl, whisk together the eggs, low·fat milk, and black pepper. Set aside.

3. Heat the olive oil in a 9·inch oven·safe skillet over medium heat. Add the diced bell peppers, zucchini, onion, and minced garlic. Sauté for 5·7 minutes until the vegetables are tender.

4. Pour the egg mixture over the sautéed vegetables in the skillet. Sprinkle the shredded low·fat cheese evenly over the top.

5. Transfer the skillet to the preheated oven and bake for 18·22 minutes, until the frittata is set and the cheese is melted.

6. Remove the frittata from the oven and let it cool for 5 minutes before slicing and serving.

This vegetable frittata is a great option for a renal diet. Eggs provide high·quality protein, while the vegetables add fiber, vitamins, and minerals. The use of low·fat cheese keeps the saturated fat and sodium content low. It's a nutritious and satisfying meal for seniors.

67. Egg white omelet with spinach and tomatoes

Ingredient:

- 4 egg whites
- 1/4 cup diced tomatoes
- 1/2 cup fresh spinach, chopped
- 1 tablespoon low•fat milk
- 1 tablespoon grated Parmesan cheese (optional)
- Salt and pepper to taste

Instructions:

1. In a small bowl, whisk together the egg whites and milk until well combined.

2. Spray a non•stick skillet with cooking spray and heat over medium heat.

3. Pour the egg white mixture into the skillet and let it cook for 2•3 minutes, or until the bottom is set.

4. Sprinkle the diced tomatoes and chopped spinach over the top of the egg whites. Using a spatula, gently fold the omelet in half and slide it onto a plate.

5. If using, sprinkle the grated Parmesan cheese over the top of the omelet. Season with a pinch of salt and pepper.

Nutritional Considerations for a Renal Diet:

- Egg whites are a high•quality protein source that is low in phosphorus, making them a great choice for those with kidney disease.

- Spinach is a good source of vitamins and minerals, but it is also high in potassium, so portion size is important.

- Tomatoes are low in potassium and phosphorus, making them a kidney•friendly vegetable.

- Low•fat milk and Parmesan cheese provide a small amount of calcium and protein without adding excessive sodium or phosphorus.

This egg white omelet with spinach and tomatoes is a nutritious and flavorful option for seniors following a renal diet. The combination of lean protein, vegetables, and a small amount of dairy makes it a balanced and satisfying meal.

68. Deviled eggs with low•sodium ingredients

Ingredient:

- 6 hard•boiled eggs
- 2 tbsp low•fat mayonnaise
- 1 tsp Dijon mustard
- 1 tsp white vinegar
- 1/4 tsp garlic powder
- 1/4 tsp paprika
- Black pepper to taste
- Chopped chives or parsley for garnish (optional)

Instructions:

1. Peel the hard•boiled eggs and cut them in half lengthwise.

2. Carefully remove the yolks and place them in a small bowl.

3. In the bowl with the yolks, mash them with a fork. Add the low•fat mayonnaise, Dijon mustard, white vinegar, garlic powder, and a pinch of black pepper. Stir until well combined.

4. Spoon or pipe the yolk mixture back into the egg white halves.

5. Sprinkle the deviled eggs with paprika.

6. Garnish with chopped chives or parsley, if desired.

7. Refrigerate the deviled eggs until ready to serve.

These deviled eggs are a great low•sodium option for a renal diet. The use of low•fat mayonnaise and Dijon mustard instead of regular mayonnaise and mustard helps reduce the sodium content. The vinegar and spices add flavor without the need for added salt. Deviled eggs are a protein•rich, bite•sized snack or appetizer that seniors on a renal diet can enjoy.

69. Quiche with spinach and mushrooms (low·fat crust)

Ingredient:

- 1 cup whole wheat flour
- 2 tablespoons cold unsalted butter, cubed
- 2·3 tablespoons ice water

Filling Ingredients:
- 6 large eggs
- 1 cup low·fat milk
- 1/4 cup grated Parmesan cheese
- 1/4 teaspoon ground nutmeg
- Salt and pepper to taste
- 1 cup fresh spinach, chopped
- 1 cup sliced mushrooms
- 1/4 cup diced onion

Instructions:

1. Make the crust:
   - In a food processor, pulse the flour and butter until mixture resembles coarse crumbs.
   - Add ice water 1 tablespoon at a time, pulsing until dough just begins to hold together.
   - Shape dough into a disk, wrap in plastic, and refrigerate for at least 30 minutes.

2. Preheat oven to 375°F (190°C).

3. Roll out the chilled dough and press it into a 9·inch pie plate. Crimp the edges decoratively.

4. In a large bowl, whisk together the eggs, milk, Parmesan, nutmeg, salt, and pepper.

5. Spread the spinach, mushrooms, and onion evenly in the prepared pie crust.

6. Pour the egg mixture over the vegetables.

7. Bake for 35·40 minutes, or until the center is set and the crust is golden brown. Allow the quiche to cool for 10 minutes before slicing and serving.

The whole wheat flour in the crust provides more fiber and nutrients compared to a traditional pie crust. The low·fat milk and minimal cheese in the filling keep this quiche light and healthy, while the spinach and mushrooms add flavor and nutrients.

70. Huevos rancheros with salsa (low·sodium)

Ingredient:

• 4 eggs
• 2 corn tortillas
• 1/2 cup low·sodium black beans, rinsed and drained
• 1/4 cup diced tomatoes
• 2 tablespoons diced onion
• 1 tablespoon chopped cilantro
• 1 teaspoon lime juice
• 1/4 teaspoon ground cumin
• Salt and pepper to taste

Low·Sodium Salsa:
• 1 cup diced tomatoes
• 2 tablespoons diced onion
• 1 tablespoon chopped cilantro
• 1 teaspoon lime juice
• 1/4 teaspoon ground cumin
• 1/8 teaspoon garlic powder
• Salt and pepper to taste

Instructions:
1. Make the low·sodium salsa by combining all the salsa ingredients in a small bowl. Season with a pinch of salt and pepper. Set aside.

2. In a small bowl, mix together the black beans, diced tomatoes, onion, cilantro, lime juice, and cumin. Season with a pinch of salt and pepper.

3. Heat a non·stick skillet over medium heat. Crack the eggs into the skillet and cook until the whites are set but the yolks are still runny, about 3·4 minutes.

4. Meanwhile, warm the corn tortillas according to package instructions.

5. To assemble, place the warm tortillas on a plate and top each one with half of the black bean mixture. Top with the cooked eggs.

6. Spoon the low·sodium salsa over the top of the eggs and serve immediately.

The key to keeping this dish low in sodium is using low·sodium black beans, limiting added salt, and making a fresh, homemade salsa without high·sodium ingredients. This makes it a healthier option for those on a renal diet.

71. Herbal teas (non•caffeinated)

Ingredient:

• 1 teaspoon dried chamomile flowers
• 1 cup (8 oz) hot water

Instructions:

1. Bring the water to a boil in a small saucepan or kettle.

2. Place the dried chamomile flowers in a tea infuser, tea ball, or directly into a mug.

3. Pour the hot water over the chamomile.

4. Allow the tea to steep for 5•7 minutes, or to your desired strength.

5. Remove the tea infuser or strain the tea to remove the chamomile flowers.

6. You can optionally add a little honey or lemon to taste.

Tips:
• Use fresh, high•quality dried chamomile flowers for the best flavor.
• Adjust the amount of chamomile to your personal preference • 1•2 teaspoons per cup is typical.
• Steep the tea for longer if you want a stronger, more potent flavor.
• Drink chamomile tea hot, as the heat helps release the beneficial compounds.

Chamomile tea is known for its calming and soothing properties. It can be enjoyed any time of day, but is especially nice before bedtime to help promote relaxation and sleep.

This simple homemade chamomile tea is a great way to enjoy the natural benefits of this herbal tea. Sip and savor the delicate, floral flavor.

72. Infused water (cucumber, lemon, mint)

Ingredient:

- 1 cucumber, sliced
- 1 lemon, sliced
- 10•12 fresh mint leaves
- 8 cups cold water

Instructions:

1. In a large pitcher or water dispenser, combine the sliced cucumber, lemon slices, and fresh mint leaves.

2. Pour the cold water over the fruit and herbs.

3. Stir gently to combine.

4. Refrigerate the infused water for at least 2 hours, or up to 8 hours, to allow the flavors to infuse.

5. Serve the cucumber, lemon, and mint infused water chilled.

This infused water is an excellent choice for seniors on a renal diet. It provides hydration without any added sugars, sweeteners, or sodium. The cucumber, lemon, and mint add natural flavor and aroma, making it a refreshing and appealing beverage.

The benefits of this infused water include:

- Hydration: Water is essential for kidney health and overall well•being.

- Low sodium: No added salts or sodium•containing ingredients.

- Antioxidants: Cucumber and lemon provide vitamins and antioxidants.

- Freshness: The mint leaves add a crisp, cooling element.

This infused water can be enjoyed throughout the day to help seniors stay hydrated while adhering to a renal•friendly diet.

73. Low·sodium vegetable juice

Ingredient:

- 2 cups chopped tomatoes
- 1 cup chopped carrots
- 1 cup chopped celery
- 1/2 cup chopped green bell pepper
- 1/4 cup chopped onion
- 2 cloves garlic, minced
- 1 cup water
- 1 tbsp lemon juice
- 1/4 tsp black pepper

Instructions:

1. In a blender, combine the chopped tomatoes, carrots, celery, bell pepper, onion, and garlic.

2. Add the water and lemon juice. Blend on high speed until smooth.

3. Pour the juice through a fine mesh strainer to remove any pulp or solids.

4. Stir in the black pepper.

5. Serve chilled or over ice.

This vegetable juice is low in sodium since it doesn't contain any added salt. The vegetables provide vitamins, minerals, and antioxidants. Adjust the amounts of each vegetable to your taste preferences. Enjoy!

74. Freshly squeezed fruit juices (in moderation)

Ingredient:

• 1 cup fresh orange juice
• 1/2 cup unsweetened almond milk
• 1/2 banana
• 1 tbsp honey (optional)
• Ice cubes

This smoothie provides vitamin C from the orange juice, while the almond milk and banana add creaminess without too much potassium.

Ginger Orange Spritzer:
• 1 cup fresh orange juice
• 1/2 cup sparkling water
• 1 tsp grated fresh ginger
• Squeeze of lemon juice
• Ice cubes

The ginger adds a nice zing, while the sparkling water makes it a refreshing spritzer. The lemon juice helps balance the sweetness.

Orange Pineapple Slush:
• 1 cup fresh orange juice
• 1/2 cup pineapple juice
• 1 tbsp lime juice
• 1 cup crushed ice

This icy treat combines citrus flavors for a tasty and hydrating option.

The key things to note for a renal·friendly orange juice recipe are:
• Use fresh, unsweetened orange juice
• Limit portion sizes to 1 cup or less
• Combine with other low·potassium ingredients like almond milk, ginger, or pineapple
• Avoid added sugars

I hope these give you some healthy and delicious orange juice ideas for your senior clients on a renal diet!

75. Smoothies with low·potassium fruits and low·fat yogurt

Ingredient:

- 1 cup low·fat plain Greek yogurt
- 1/2 cup unsweetened almond milk (or low·fat milk)
- 1/2 cup blueberries
- 1/2 cup strawberries
- 1 tablespoon honey (optional)
- 1/2 teaspoon vanilla extract

Instructions:

1. Add the yogurt, almond milk, blueberries, strawberries, honey (if using), and vanilla extract to a blender.

2. Blend on high speed until smooth and creamy, about 1 minute. Pour the smoothie into a glass and enjoy immediately.

Nutritional Considerations for a Renal Diet:

- Low·fat plain Greek yogurt is a great source of protein without excessive phosphorus or potassium.
- Blueberries and strawberries are lower in potassium compared to many other fruits, making them a good choice for those on a renal diet.
- Almond milk is low in potassium and phosphorus, providing a dairy·free alternative to regular milk.
- Honey can be used in moderation to add sweetness without impacting electrolyte levels.

Tips:
- You can use any combination of low·potassium fruits like raspberries, blackberries, or pineapple.
- Add a handful of spinach or kale for extra nutrients, but be mindful of the potassium content.
- For a thicker smoothie, use frozen fruit instead of fresh.
- Adjust the amount of honey or milk to reach your desired consistency and sweetness.

This low·potassium fruit smoothie is a refreshing and nutritious option for those following a renal diet. The combination of low·fat yogurt and low·potassium fruits provides a satisfying and kidney·friendly treat.

76. Farro salad with vegetables and vinaigrette

Ingredient:

- 1 cup dry farro, cooked according to package instructions and cooled
- 1 cup diced cucumber
- 1 cup cherry tomatoes, halved
- 1/2 cup diced bell pepper
- 1/4 cup diced red onion
- 2 tbsp chopped fresh parsley
- 2 tbsp olive oil
- 1 tbsp white wine vinegar
- 1 tsp Dijon mustard
- 1 tsp honey
- Salt and pepper to taste

Instructions:

1. In a large bowl, combine the cooked and cooled farro, cucumber, tomatoes, bell pepper, red onion, and parsley.

2. In a small bowl, whisk together the olive oil, vinegar, Dijon, and honey. Season with a pinch of salt and pepper.

3. Pour the vinaigrette over the farro salad and toss gently to coat.

4. Serve chilled or at room temperature.

This farro salad is a great option for seniors on a renal diet as it is:
- Low in potassium from the vegetables
- High in fiber from the farro
- Light and refreshing with the vinaigrette
- Easy to prepare and enjoy

The farro provides complex carbs and protein, while the veggies add vitamins, minerals and antioxidants. Feel free to adjust the vegetable mix to your preference. Enjoy!

77. Buckwheat pancakes with low•sodium syrup

Ingredient:

- 1 cup buckwheat flour
- 1 tsp baking powder
- 1/4 tsp salt
- 1 egg
- 1 cup unsweetened almond milk
- 1 tbsp honey
- 1 tsp vanilla extract

Low•Sodium Syrup Ingredients:
- 1/2 cup unsweetened apple juice
- 1 tbsp honey
- 1/2 tsp ground cinnamon

Instructions:

1. In a medium bowl, whisk together the buckwheat flour, baking powder, and salt.

2. In a separate bowl, beat the egg. Then whisk in the almond milk, honey, and vanilla.

3. Pour the wet ingredients into the dry ingredients and stir just until combined (do not overmix).

4. Heat a lightly oiled skillet or griddle over medium heat. Scoop the batter onto the hot surface, using about 1/4 cup per pancake.

5. Cook for 2•3 minutes per side, until golden brown.

6. For the low•sodium syrup, combine the apple juice, honey, and cinnamon in a small saucepan. Warm over low heat, stirring occasionally, until heated through.

7. Serve the buckwheat pancakes warm, drizzled with the low•sodium cinnamon•apple syrup.

These buckwheat pancakes are a great option for seniors on a renal diet as they are:
- Low in sodium from the lack of added salt
- Lower in potassium than traditional pancakes
- High in fiber from the buckwheat flour
- Sweetened with honey instead of sugar

78. Couscous with roasted vegetables

Ingredient:

- 1 cup dry whole wheat couscous
- 1 1/4 cups low•sodium vegetable or chicken broth
- 1 medium zucchini, diced
- 1 red bell pepper, diced
- 1 cup cherry tomatoes, halved
- 1 small red onion, diced
- 2 tbsp olive oil
- 1 tbsp lemon juice
- 2 tbsp chopped fresh parsley
- Salt and pepper to taste

Instructions:

1. Preheat oven to 400°F. Toss the diced zucchini, bell pepper, and onion with 1 tbsp of the olive oil on a baking sheet. Roast for 20•25 minutes, until vegetables are tender and lightly browned.

2. Meanwhile, bring the vegetable or chicken broth to a boil in a medium saucepan. Remove from heat, stir in the couscous, cover and let sit for 5•7 minutes until couscous is tender.

3. Fluff the cooked couscous with a fork and transfer to a large bowl.

4. Add the roasted vegetables, cherry tomatoes, remaining 1 tbsp olive oil, lemon juice, and chopped parsley. Toss gently to combine.

5. Season the couscous salad with a pinch of salt and pepper to taste.

6. Serve the couscous with roasted vegetables warm or chilled.

This couscous salad is a great option for seniors on a renal diet as:

- Couscous is low in sodium and potassium
- The roasted vegetables add fiber, vitamins and minerals without too much potassium
- The lemon juice and parsley provide flavor without added salt

Feel free to adjust the vegetable mix based on your preferences. This makes a tasty and nutritious side dish or light main course. Enjoy!

79. Millet pilaf with herbs

Ingredient:

- 1 cup dry millet, rinsed
- 2 cups low•sodium vegetable or chicken broth
- 2 tbsp olive oil
- 1 small onion, diced
- 2 cloves garlic, minced
- 1/4 cup chopped fresh parsley
- 2 tbsp chopped fresh thyme
- 2 tbsp chopped fresh basil
- Salt and pepper to taste

Instructions:

1. In a medium saucepan, bring the millet and broth to a boil over high heat. Once boiling, reduce heat to low, cover and simmer for 20•25 minutes, until millet is tender and liquid is absorbed.

2. While the millet is cooking, heat the olive oil in a skillet over medium heat. Add the diced onion and sauté for 5•7 minutes until translucent.

3. Add the minced garlic and sauté for 1 minute more, until fragrant.

4. Fluff the cooked millet with a fork and stir in the sautéed onions and garlic.

5. Fold in the chopped parsley, thyme, and basil. Season with a pinch of salt and pepper to taste.

6. Serve the millet pilaf warm, garnished with extra fresh herbs if desired.

This millet pilaf is a great option for seniors on a renal diet as:

- Millet is low in sodium and potassium
- The fresh herbs add flavor without added salt
- It's a simple, plant•based side dish that's easy to prepare

Millet is a gluten•free whole grain that provides fiber, protein, and B vitamins. Feel free to adjust the herb blend to your taste preferences. Enjoy this flavorful and nutritious pilaf!

80. Whole wheat bread with low•sodium spreads

Ingredient:

- 2 cups whole wheat flour
- 1 tsp baking powder
- 1/2 tsp baking soda
- 1/4 tsp salt
- 1 cup unsweetened almond milk
- 2 tbsp honey
- 1 tbsp olive oil

Low•Sodium Spread Options:
- Avocado mash
- Hummus
- Nut butter (peanut, almond, cashew)
- Cream cheese with fresh herbs
- Olive oil and balsamic vinegar

Instructions:

1. Preheat oven to 375°F. Grease a 9x5 inch loaf pan.

2. In a large bowl, whisk together the whole wheat flour, baking powder, baking soda, and salt.

3. In a separate bowl, combine the almond milk, honey, and olive oil.

4. Pour the wet ingredients into the dry ingredients and stir just until combined (do not overmix).

5. Transfer the batter to the prepared loaf pan and bake for 30•35 minutes, until a toothpick inserted in the center comes out clean.

6. Allow the bread to cool completely before slicing. Serve slices of the whole wheat bread with your choice of low•sodium spread.

Some tasty low•sodium spread ideas:
- Mash up a ripe avocado and season with a squeeze of lemon juice
- Spread hummus made with low•sodium chickpeas
- Use natural nut butters without added salt
- Mix cream cheese with chopped fresh herbs like parsley or basil
- Drizzle with olive oil and balsamic vinegar

81. Chicken and rice casserole with vegetables

Ingredient:

- 1 cup uncooked brown rice
- 1 lb boneless, skinless chicken breasts, cubed
- 1 cup diced carrots
- 1 cup diced zucchini
- 1/2 cup diced onion
- 1 cup low•sodium chicken broth
- 1 tbsp olive oil
- 1 tsp dried thyme
- 1/2 tsp garlic powder
- Salt and pepper to taste

Instructions:

1. Preheat oven to 375°F. Grease a 9x13 inch baking dish.

2. Cook the brown rice according to package instructions. Set aside.

3. In a large skillet, heat the olive oil over medium heat. Add the diced chicken and sauté for 5•7 minutes until lightly browned.

4. Add the diced carrots, zucchini, and onion to the skillet. Sauté for 3•4 minutes until vegetables start to soften.

5. Transfer the chicken and vegetable mixture to the prepared baking dish.

6. Stir in the cooked brown rice and chicken broth. Season with the thyme, garlic powder, salt and pepper.

7. Cover the dish with foil and bake for 30•35 minutes, until the rice is tender and the chicken is cooked through.

8. Remove the foil and let the casserole cool for 5 minutes before serving.

This chicken and rice casserole is a great option for seniors on a renal diet as:

- Brown rice is low in sodium and potassium
- The vegetables add fiber and nutrients without too much potassium
- It's a one•dish meal that's easy to prepare

82. Eggplant lasagna (low•fat cheese)

Ingredient:

- 1 teaspoon dried oregano
- 1/2 teaspoon dried basil
- Salt and pepper to taste
- 1 cup part•skim ricotta cheese
- 1 egg
- 1/4 cup grated Parmesan cheese
- 1 cup shredded part•skim mozzarella cheese

- 2 medium eggplants, sliced lengthwise into 1/4•inch thick slices
- 1 tablespoon olive oil
- 1 onion, diced
- 3 cloves garlic, minced
- 1 (28 oz) can crushed tomatoes

Instructions:

1. Preheat your oven to 375°F (190°C).

2. Brush the eggplant slices lightly with olive oil and place them on a baking sheet. Roast for 15•20 minutes, flipping halfway, until tender.

3. In a large skillet, heat the remaining 1 tablespoon of olive oil over medium heat. Add the diced onion and minced garlic. Sauté for 3•5 minutes until the onion is translucent.

4. Add the crushed tomatoes, oregano, basil, salt, and pepper. Simmer the sauce for 10•15 minutes, stirring occasionally.

5. In a small bowl, mix together the ricotta cheese, egg, and Parmesan cheese.

6. Spread a thin layer of the tomato sauce in the bottom of a 9x13 inch baking dish. Arrange a layer of the roasted eggplant slices over the sauce. Spread half of the ricotta cheese mixture over the eggplant, then top with 1/3 of the mozzarella cheese.

7. Repeat the layers of eggplant, ricotta, and mozzarella cheese. Top with the remaining tomato sauce and mozzarella cheese.

8. Bake the lasagna for 30•35 minutes, or until the cheese is melted and bubbly. Let the lasagna cool for 10•15 minutes before serving.

This eggplant lasagna uses low•fat cheeses to reduce the overall fat and calorie content, making it a healthier option. The roasted eggplant slices replace the traditional pasta layers, creating a delicious and nutritious dish.

83. Quinoa and vegetable bake

Ingredient:

- 1 cup dry quinoa, rinsed
- 2 cups low•sodium vegetable or chicken broth
- 1 tbsp olive oil
- 1 onion, diced
- 2 cloves garlic, minced
- 1 cup diced zucchini
- 1 cup diced bell pepper
- 1 cup diced mushrooms
- 1 (15 oz) can low•sodium diced tomatoes
- 2 tbsp chopped fresh basil
- 1 tsp dried oregano
- Salt and pepper to taste
- 1/4 cup shredded low•sodium mozzarella cheese (optional)

Instructions:

1. Preheat oven to 375°F. Grease an 8x8 inch baking dish.

2. In a medium saucepan, combine the quinoa and broth. Bring to a boil, then reduce heat and simmer for 15•20 minutes, until quinoa is tender. Fluff with a fork.

3. In a skillet, heat the olive oil over medium heat. Add the diced onion and sauté for 5 minutes until translucent.

4. Add the minced garlic, zucchini, bell pepper, and mushrooms. Sauté for 3•4 minutes more until vegetables are tender.

5. Transfer the cooked quinoa to a large bowl. Stir in the sautéed vegetables, diced tomatoes, chopped basil, and oregano. Season with a pinch of salt and pepper.

6. Spread the quinoa and vegetable mixture evenly into the prepared baking dish.

7. If using, sprinkle the shredded mozzarella cheese over the top.

8. Bake for 20•25 minutes, until heated through and cheese is melted. Let stand for 5 minutes before serving.

Feel free to adjust the vegetable blend based on your preferences. Enjoy this nutritious and flavorful bake!

84. Lentil and brown rice casserole

Ingredient:

- 1 cup dry brown rice, cooked according to package
- 1 cup dry brown lentils, rinsed
- 4 cups low•sodium vegetable or chicken broth
- 1 tbsp olive oil
- 1 onion, diced
- 2 carrots, peeled and diced
- 2 celery stalks, diced
- 3 cloves garlic, minced
- 1 tsp dried thyme
- 1/2 tsp dried oregano
- Salt and pepper to taste

Instructions:

1. Preheat oven to 375°F. Grease a 9x13 inch baking dish.

2. In a large saucepan, combine the lentils and broth. Bring to a boil, then reduce heat and simmer for 20•25 minutes, until lentils are tender. Drain any excess liquid.

3. In a skillet, heat the olive oil over medium heat. Add the diced onion, carrots, and celery. Sauté for 5•7 minutes until vegetables are softened.

4. Stir the cooked vegetables into the cooked lentils. Add the minced garlic, thyme, oregano, and a pinch of salt and pepper.

5. Fold in the cooked brown rice until everything is well combined.

6. Transfer the lentil and rice mixture to the prepared baking dish.

7. Bake for 25•30 minutes, until heated through.

8. Let the casserole cool for 5 minutes before serving.

Feel free to adjust the vegetable blend to your preference. Serve this casserole on its own or with a simple green salad. Enjoy!

85. Potato and green bean casserole (low·fat)

Ingredient:

- 2 lbs russet potatoes, peeled and cut into 1·inch cubes
- 1 lb fresh green beans, trimmed and cut into 1·inch pieces
- 1 onion, diced
- 2 cloves garlic, minced
- 1 cup low·sodium chicken or vegetable broth
- 2 tbsp low·fat plain Greek yogurt
- 1 tbsp Dijon mustard
- 1/4 tsp dried thyme
- Salt and pepper to taste
- 1/4 cup panko breadcrumbs
- 2 tbsp grated Parmesan cheese (optional)

Instructions:

1. Preheat oven to 375°F. Grease a 9x13 inch baking dish.

2. In a large pot, cover the potato cubes with water and bring to a boil. Cook for 5 minutes, then add the green bean pieces. Cook for 3·4 minutes more until potatoes are tender and green beans are crisp·tender. Drain and set aside.

3. In a skillet, sauté the diced onion over medium heat for 5 minutes until translucent. Add the minced garlic and cook for 1 minute more.

4. In a large bowl, combine the cooked potatoes and green beans, sautéed onions and garlic, broth, Greek yogurt, Dijon, and thyme. Season with a pinch of salt and pepper.

5. Transfer the potato and green bean mixture to the prepared baking dish. Top with the panko breadcrumbs and Parmesan cheese (if using).

6. Bake for 25·30 minutes, until the top is golden brown and the casserole is bubbling.

7. Let stand for 5 minutes before serving.

This potato and green bean casserole is a great option for seniors on a renal diet because:

- Potatoes and green beans are relatively low in potassium
- The Greek yogurt provides creaminess without excess fat or sodium
- Panko breadcrumbs add a crispy topping without much sodium

86. Caprese salad skewers (low•sodium cheese)

Ingredient:

• 8 oz low•sodium mozzarella cheese, cut into 1•inch cubes
• 1 pint cherry or grape tomatoes
• 16•20 fresh basil leaves
• 2 tbsp balsamic glaze
• 1 tbsp olive oil
• Freshly ground black pepper

Equipment:
• 8•10 wooden or metal skewers

Instructions:

1. Thread the mozzarella cubes, tomatoes, and basil leaves onto the skewers, alternating the ingredients.

2. Arrange the caprese skewers on a serving platter.

3. Drizzle the balsamic glaze and olive oil over the skewers.

4. Finish with a light sprinkle of freshly ground black pepper.

5. Serve immediately or chill until ready to serve.

These caprese salad skewers are a great option for seniors on a renal diet for a few reasons:

• Low•sodium mozzarella cheese keeps the sodium content down
• Tomatoes and basil are low in potassium
• The balsamic glaze and olive oil provide flavor without added salt
• The portion size is controlled with the skewers

The combination of the creamy mozzarella, juicy tomatoes, and fresh basil makes for a refreshing and flavorful appetizer or snack. Feel free to use cherry tomatoes or grape tomatoes based on your preference.

This is a simple, no•cook recipe that's easy to prepare and enjoy. Serve these caprese skewers at your next gathering or as a light bite. Enjoy!

87. Stuffed mushrooms with spinach and feta

Ingredient:

- 12 oz cremini or button mushrooms, stems removed and finely chopped
- 1 tbsp olive oil
- 1/2 cup chopped fresh spinach
- 2 oz crumbled low•sodium feta cheese
- 1 tbsp chopped fresh parsley
- 1 clove garlic, minced
- 1/4 tsp dried oregano
- Salt and pepper to taste

Instructions:

1. Preheat oven to 375°F. Lightly grease a baking sheet.

2. Gently wipe the mushroom caps clean with a damp paper towel. Carefully remove the stems and finely chop them.

3. In a skillet, heat the olive oil over medium heat. Add the chopped mushroom stems, spinach, garlic, oregano, and a pinch of salt and pepper. Sauté for 3•4 minutes until the spinach is wilted.

4. Remove the skillet from heat and stir in the crumbled feta cheese and chopped parsley.

5. Spoon the spinach•feta filling into the mushroom caps, dividing it evenly.

6. Arrange the stuffed mushrooms on the prepared baking sheet.

7. Bake for 12•15 minutes, until the mushrooms are tender and the filling is hot.

8. Serve the stuffed mushrooms warm.

The combination of the savory filling and tender mushroom caps makes for a tasty and satisfying appetizer. Feel free to adjust the herb and seasoning blend to your taste preferences.

This is a simple, no•fuss recipe that's easy to prepare. Enjoy these stuffed mushrooms as a healthy snack or appetizer!

88. Cucumber and tomato bruschetta

Ingredient:

- 1 baguette, sliced into 1/2•inch thick rounds
- 2 tbsp olive oil
- 1 cup diced cucumber
- 1 cup diced tomatoes
- 2 tbsp chopped fresh basil
- 1 tbsp balsamic vinegar
- 1 clove garlic, minced
- Salt and pepper to taste

Instructions:

1. Preheat oven to 400°F. Arrange the baguette slices on a baking sheet and brush lightly with 1 tbsp of the olive oil. Bake for 5•7 minutes until lightly toasted.

2. In a medium bowl, combine the diced cucumber, tomatoes, basil, balsamic vinegar, garlic, and remaining 1 tbsp olive oil. Season with a pinch of salt and pepper.

3. Top each toasted baguette slice with a spoonful of the cucumber•tomato mixture.

4. Serve the bruschetta immediately, while the bread is still warm and crisp.

This cucumber and tomato bruschetta is a great option for seniors on a renal diet for a few reasons:

- The vegetables (cucumber and tomato) are low in potassium

- There is minimal added salt, with just a pinch to season

- The balsamic vinegar and fresh basil provide flavor without sodium

- The portion size is controlled with the baguette slices

The combination of the crisp bread, juicy tomatoes, and refreshing cucumber makes for a tasty and hydrating appetizer or snack. Feel free to adjust the vegetable ratio to your preference. Enjoy!

89. Shrimp cocktail with low·sodium sauce

Ingredient:

For the Shrimp:
• 1 lb cooked, peeled and deveined shrimp, tails left on
• Lemon wedges for serving

For the Cocktail Sauce:
• 1/2 cup ketchup
• 2 tbsp lemon juice
• 1 tbsp prepared horseradish
• 1 tsp Worcestershire sauce (low·sodium if available)
• 1/4 tsp ground black pepper

Instructions:

1. In a small bowl, whisk together all the ingredients for the cocktail sauce. Taste and adjust seasoning as needed.

2. Arrange the cooked shrimp on a serving platter or in individual cocktail glasses.

3. Serve the shrimp chilled, with the low·sodium cocktail sauce on the side for dipping.

4. Garnish with lemon wedges.

This shrimp cocktail is a great option for seniors on a renal diet for a few reasons:

• Shrimp is a lean protein that's low in sodium and potassium
• The homemade cocktail sauce is low in sodium compared to store·bought versions
• The portion size is controlled, making it a light and refreshing appetizer

The key to keeping the sodium low in the cocktail sauce is to use regular ketchup instead of a low·sodium version (which can still be high in sodium) and to avoid adding extra salt.

This classic shrimp cocktail makes for an elegant and tasty start to any meal. Enjoy!

90. Roasted red pepper hummus with vegetables

Ingredient:

• 1 (15 oz) can low•sodium chickpeas, rinsed and drained
• 1/4 cup tahini
• 2 tbsp lemon juice
• 2 tbsp olive oil
• 1 roasted red pepper, chopped
• 2 cloves garlic, minced
• 1/4 tsp ground cumin
• Salt and pepper to taste

Vegetable Dippers:
• Baby carrots
• Cucumber slices
• Celery sticks
• Bell pepper strips

Instructions:

1. In a food processor, combine all the hummus ingredients. Blend until smooth and creamy, scraping down the sides as needed.

2. Taste the hummus and adjust seasoning with salt and pepper as desired.

3. Transfer the roasted red pepper hummus to a serving bowl.

4. Arrange the assorted vegetable dippers around the hummus.

5. Serve immediately, or refrigerate until ready to serve.

This roasted red pepper hummus is a great option for seniors on a renal diet for a few reasons:

• Chickpeas are low in sodium and potassium
• Roasted red peppers add flavor without extra sodium
• The vegetable dippers (carrots, cucumbers, celery, peppers) are also low in potassium
• It's a nutrient•dense, high•fiber snack or appetizer

The homemade hummus is easy to prepare and much lower in sodium than store•bought versions. Feel free to adjust the amount of garlic, lemon juice, or spices to your taste preferences.

91. Stir•fried chicken with ginger and vegetables

Ingredient:

- 1 lb boneless, skinless chicken breasts, cut into 1•inch pieces
- 2 tbsp low•sodium soy sauce
- 1 tbsp rice vinegar
- 1 tsp sesame oil
- 2 tsp grated fresh ginger
- 2 cloves garlic, minced
- 2 tbsp olive oil
- 1 cup sliced mushrooms
- 1 cup sliced bell peppers
- 1 cup snow peas or snap peas
- 2 cups cooked brown rice, for serving

Instructions:

1. In a medium bowl, combine the chicken, soy sauce, rice vinegar, sesame oil, ginger, and garlic. Toss to coat the chicken and let marinate for 15 minutes.

2. Heat the olive oil in a large skillet or wok over high heat. Add the marinated chicken and stir•fry for 5•7 minutes until cooked through.

3. Add the sliced mushrooms, bell peppers, and snow peas to the skillet. Stir•fry for an additional 3•5 minutes, until the vegetables are tender•crisp.

4. Serve the stir•fried chicken and vegetables immediately over the cooked brown rice.

This stir•fry dish is a great option for seniors on a renal diet for a few reasons:

- Chicken is a lean protein that's low in sodium and potassium
- The vegetables (mushrooms, peppers, snow peas) are also low in potassium
- Brown rice provides complex carbs and fiber without excess sodium
- The ginger, garlic, and rice vinegar add flavor without needing much added salt

Feel free to adjust the vegetable mix based on your preferences. This makes a quick, healthy, and delicious one•dish meal. Enjoy!

92. Beef and broccoli stir•fry (low•sodium sauce)

Ingredient:

- 1 lb beef sirloin or flank steak, thinly sliced
- 3 cups broccoli florets
- 2 tbsp olive oil
- 2 cloves garlic, minced
- 1 tbsp grated fresh ginger
- 1/4 cup low•sodium beef or chicken broth
- 2 tbsp low•sodium soy sauce
- 1 tbsp rice vinegar
- 1 tsp honey
- 1/4 tsp red pepper flakes (optional)
- 2 cups cooked brown rice, for serving

Instructions:

1. In a small bowl, whisk together the broth, soy sauce, rice vinegar, honey, and red pepper flakes (if using). Set aside.

2. Heat 1 tbsp of the olive oil in a large skillet or wok over high heat. Add the beef and stir•fry for 3•4 minutes until browned. Remove the beef from the pan and set aside.

3. Add the remaining 1 tbsp olive oil to the pan. Add the broccoli florets and stir•fry for 2•3 minutes until crisp•tender.

4. Push the broccoli to the sides of the pan. Add the minced garlic and grated ginger to the center and cook for 1 minute until fragrant.

5. Pour the sauce mixture into the pan and bring to a simmer. Add the cooked beef back to the pan and toss everything together until well coated in the sauce.

6. Cook for 2•3 minutes more, until the sauce has thickened slightly.

7. Serve the beef and broccoli stir•fry immediately over the cooked brown rice.

This beef and broccoli dish is a great option for seniors on a renal diet because:

- Beef is a lean protein that's low in sodium and potassium
- Broccoli is a low•potassium vegetable
- The homemade low•sodium sauce keeps the sodium content down

93. Sushi rolls with cucumber and avocado

Ingredient:

- 1 cup short•grain brown rice, cooked according to package
- 4 sheets nori (seaweed sheets)
- 1 medium cucumber, peeled, seeded and cut into thin strips
- 1 ripe avocado, sliced
- 2 tbsp rice vinegar
- 1 tsp honey
- 1 tsp sesame seeds (optional)

Equipment Needed:
- Bamboo sushi rolling mat

Instructions:

1. In a small bowl, mix together the rice vinegar and honey. Gently fold this into the cooked brown rice until well combined.

2. Lay a sheet of nori shiny•side down on the sushi mat. Spread about 1/4 cup of the seasoned rice evenly over the nori, leaving a 1•inch strip bare at the top.

3. Arrange a few strips of cucumber and a couple slices of avocado in a line across the center of the rice.

4. Starting from the bottom, use the sushi mat to tightly roll up the nori around the fillings. Moisten the bare nori strip with a bit of water to help seal the roll.

5. Repeat with the remaining nori sheets and fillings.

6. Slice each roll into 6•8 pieces using a sharp knife. Wet the knife between cuts to prevent sticking.

7. Arrange the sushi rolls on a plate and sprinkle with sesame seeds if desired.

These cucumber and avocado sushi rolls are a great option for seniors on a renal diet because:

- Brown rice is lower in potassium than white rice
- Cucumber and avocado are both low•potassium vegetables
- There is minimal added sodium, just from the rice vinegar

94. Thai coconut curry
with chicken (low•fat coconut milk)

Ingredient:

- 1 lb boneless, skinless chicken breasts, cut into 1•inch pieces
- 1 tbsp olive oil
- 1 onion, diced
- 2 cloves garlic, minced
- 1 tbsp grated fresh ginger
- 2 tsp Thai red curry paste
- 1 (13.5 oz) can low•fat coconut milk
- 1 cup low•sodium chicken broth
- 1 cup sliced mushrooms
- 1 cup sliced bell peppers
- 1 cup snow peas or snap peas
- 2 tbsp lime juice
- 2 tbsp chopped fresh cilantro
- Salt and pepper to taste
- Cooked brown rice, for serving

Instructions:

1. In a large skillet or wok, heat the olive oil over medium•high heat. Add the chicken and sauté for 5•7 minutes until lightly browned.

2. Add the diced onion, minced garlic, and grated ginger to the pan. Cook for 2•3 minutes until fragrant.

3. Stir in the Thai red curry paste and cook for 1 minute more.

4. Pour in the low•fat coconut milk and chicken broth. Bring the mixture to a simmer.

5. Add the sliced mushrooms, bell peppers, and snow peas. Simmer for 10•12 minutes, until the vegetables are tender and the chicken is cooked through.

6. Remove from heat and stir in the lime juice and chopped cilantro. Season with salt and pepper to taste. Serve the Thai coconut curry immediately over cooked brown rice.

The combination of the rich coconut curry, tender chicken, and fresh vegetables makes for a flavorful and nutritious one•dish meal. Enjoy!

95. Vegetable spring rolls with dipping sauce

Ingredient:

- 8 rice paper wrappers
- 1 cup shredded cabbage
- 1 cup shredded carrots
- 1 cup thinly sliced cucumber
- 1/2 cup thinly sliced red bell pepper
- 1/4 cup chopped fresh cilantro
- 2 tbsp chopped fresh mint

Dipping Sauce Ingredients:
- 2 tbsp low•sodium soy sauce
- 1 tbsp rice vinegar
- 1 tsp sesame oil
- 1 tsp honey
- 1 tsp grated fresh ginger
- 1 clove garlic, minced
- 1/4 tsp red pepper flakes (optional)

Instructions:

1. In a small bowl, whisk together all the dipping sauce ingredients. Set aside.

2. Fill a shallow dish with warm water. Working with one rice paper wrapper at a time, submerge it in the water for 10•15 seconds until softened.

3. Transfer the softened wrapper to a clean, damp surface. Place a small amount of the shredded cabbage, carrots, cucumber, bell pepper, cilantro, and mint in the center.

4. Fold the bottom of the wrapper up over the filling, then fold in the sides and continue rolling up tightly to enclose the filling.

5. Place the completed spring roll seam•side down on a serving platter. Repeat with the remaining wrappers and fillings.

6. Serve the fresh spring rolls immediately with the low•sodium dipping sauce on the side.

The combination of the crisp, fresh veggies and the flavorful yet low•sodium dipping sauce makes for a tasty and hydrating snack or appetizer. Enjoy!

96. Chicken enchiladas
with green sauce (low•sodium)

Ingredient:

For the Enchiladas:
• 2 cups shredded cooked chicken breast
• 8 small corn tortillas
• 1 cup shredded low•sodium Monterey Jack cheese

For the Green Sauce:
• 1 lb tomatillos, husks removed and rinsed
• 1 jalapeño, seeded and chopped
• 1 clove garlic, minced
• 1/4 cup low•sodium chicken broth
• 2 tbsp chopped fresh cilantro
• 1 tbsp lime juice
• 1/4 tsp ground cumin
• Salt and pepper to taste

Instructions:

1. Preheat oven to 375°F. Grease a 9x13 inch baking dish.

2. Make the green sauce: In a blender or food processor, combine the tomatillos, jalapeño, garlic, chicken broth, cilantro, lime juice, and cumin. Blend until smooth. Season with a pinch of salt and pepper.

3. Spread 1/2 cup of the green sauce in the bottom of the prepared baking dish.

4. Place about 1/4 cup of the shredded chicken down the center of each corn tortilla. Roll up the tortilla and place seam•side down in the baking dish.

5. Pour the remaining green sauce over the enchiladas, making sure to cover them completely. Sprinkle the shredded Monterey Jack cheese over the top.

7. Bake for 20•25 minutes, until the cheese is melted and the sauce is bubbling. Let the enchiladas cool for 5 minutes before serving.

This makes a comforting and flavorful Mexican•inspired meal. Serve it with a simple side salad for a complete renal•friendly dinner. Enjoy!

97. Bean and cheese burritos (low·sodium beans)

Ingredient:

- 1 (15 oz) can low·sodium pinto beans, rinsed and drained
- 1 tsp olive oil
- 1 clove garlic, minced
- 1 tsp ground cumin
- 1/4 tsp chili powder
- Salt and pepper to taste
- 6 large whole wheat tortillas
- 3/4 cup shredded low·sodium cheddar or Monterey Jack cheese
- Chopped fresh cilantro (optional)

Instructions:

1. In a medium saucepan, heat the olive oil over medium heat. Add the minced garlic and sauté for 1 minute until fragrant.

2. Add the rinsed and drained pinto beans, cumin, chili powder, and a pinch of salt and pepper. Mash the beans slightly with a fork or potato masher, leaving some texture.

3. Cook the bean mixture for 3·4 minutes, stirring frequently, until heated through.

4. Warm the whole wheat tortillas according to package instructions.

5. Spread about 1/3 cup of the seasoned bean mixture down the center of each tortilla.

6. Top the beans with 2·3 tablespoons of the shredded low·sodium cheese.

7. Fold the bottom of the tortilla up over the filling, then fold in the sides and continue rolling up to enclose the filling.

8. Place the burritos seam·side down on a plate. Top with chopped fresh cilantro if desired.

9. Serve the bean and cheese burritos immediately.

Feel free to adjust the spices or add any other low·potassium veggie fillings you prefer. Enjoy these tasty and nutritious burritos!

98. Grilled fish tacos with cabbage slaw

Ingredient:

For the Fish:
• 1 lb white fish fillets (such as tilapia, cod or halibut)
• 1 tbsp olive oil
• 1 tsp chili powder
• 1/2 tsp cumin
• Salt and pepper to taste

For the Cabbage Slaw:
• 2 cups shredded green cabbage
• 1 cup shredded red cabbage
• 1/4 cup chopped fresh cilantro
• 2 tbsp lime juice
• 1 tbsp olive oil
• 1/4 tsp salt

For Serving:
• 8•10 small corn tortillas, warmed
• Lime wedges

Instructions:
1. Preheat grill or grill pan to medium•high heat.

2. In a small bowl, mix together the olive oil, chili powder, cumin, salt and pepper. Rub this seasoning mixture all over the fish fillets.

3. Grill the fish for 3•4 minutes per side, until cooked through and flaky.

4. In a medium bowl, toss together the shredded green and red cabbage, cilantro, lime juice, olive oil and salt for the slaw.

5. Flake the grilled fish into bite•sized pieces.

6. To assemble the tacos, place some of the fish in the center of each warm corn tortilla. Top with a spoonful of the cabbage slaw.

7. Serve the fish tacos immediately, with lime wedges on the side.

This makes a light, flavorful and nutritious meal. Feel free to adjust the vegetable blend in the slaw to your preference. Enjoy these tasty fish tacos!

99. Guacamole with low•sodium tortilla chips

Ingredient:

- 3 ripe avocados, pitted and diced
- 1/4 cup diced red onion
- 2 tbsp chopped fresh cilantro
- 1 tbsp lime juice
- 1 clove garlic, minced
- 1/4 tsp ground cumin
- Salt and pepper to taste

Tortilla Chips:
- 8 oz low•sodium corn tortilla chips

Instructions:

1. In a medium bowl, gently mix together the diced avocado, red onion, cilantro, lime juice, garlic, and cumin.

2. Mash about half of the avocado mixture with a fork, leaving the other half in larger chunks.

3. Season the guacamole with a pinch of salt and pepper to taste.

4. Serve the guacamole immediately with the low•sodium tortilla chips on the side.

This guacamole is a great option for seniors on a renal diet for a few reasons:

- Avocados are low in sodium and potassium
- The other ingredients (onion, cilantro, lime) add flavor without much added salt
- Low•sodium tortilla chips keep the sodium content down

The combination of the creamy, flavorful guacamole and the crunchy, lightly salted tortilla chips makes for a satisfying and nutritious snack or appetizer.

Be sure to use low•sodium tortilla chips, as regular chips can be very high in sodium. You can also serve the guacamole with fresh veggie dippers like carrot sticks or cucumber slices for an even healthier option.

Enjoy this tasty and renal•friendly guacamole and chip combo!

100. Fajitas with lean beef or chicken

Ingredient:

• 1 lb lean beef sirloin or chicken breasts, thinly sliced
• 2 tbsp olive oil
• 1 onion, thinly sliced
• 2 bell peppers, thinly sliced
• 2 tsp chili powder
• 1 tsp ground cumin
• 1/2 tsp garlic powder
• Salt and pepper to taste
• 8•10 small whole wheat tortillas, warmed
• Toppings: diced tomatoes, shredded lettuce, low•sodium salsa, lime wedges

Instructions:

1. In a large skillet or wok, heat the olive oil over high heat.

2. Add the sliced beef or chicken and sauté for 3•4 minutes until lightly browned.

3. Add the sliced onions and bell peppers. Continue stir•frying for 5•7 minutes until the vegetables are tender•crisp.

4. Sprinkle the chili powder, cumin, garlic powder, and a pinch of salt and pepper over the meat and vegetables. Toss to coat evenly.

5. Serve the fajita filling immediately, with the warmed whole wheat tortillas and desired toppings on the side.

6. Let guests assemble their own fajitas by spooning the meat and veggie mixture into the tortillas and adding their choice of toppings.

These fajitas are a great option for seniors on a renal diet for a few reasons:

• Lean beef or chicken are low in sodium and potassium
• Bell peppers and onions are also low in potassium
• Whole wheat tortillas are higher in fiber than flour tortillas
• The simple spice blend adds flavor without much added salt

The customizable nature of fajitas allows seniors to control their portions and toppings to meet their dietary needs. Serve with a side salad or low•sodium rice for a complete meal.

101. Chicken piccata with lemon sauce

Ingredient:

- 1 lb boneless, skinless chicken breasts, pounded thin
- 2 tbsp all•purpose flour
- 2 tbsp olive oil
- 1/4 cup low•sodium chicken broth
- 2 tbsp fresh lemon juice
- 1 tbsp capers, rinsed
- 2 tbsp chopped fresh parsley
- Salt and pepper to taste
- Lemon wedges for serving

Instructions:

1. Season the pounded chicken breasts with a pinch of salt and pepper.

2. Dredge the chicken in the all•purpose flour, shaking off any excess.

3. In a large skillet, heat the olive oil over medium•high heat.

4. Add the floured chicken breasts and cook for 3•4 minutes per side until golden brown and cooked through. Transfer the chicken to a plate and cover to keep warm.

5. In the same skillet, add the low•sodium chicken broth and lemon juice. Bring the sauce to a simmer, scraping up any browned bits from the bottom of the pan.

6. Stir in the rinsed capers and chopped parsley. Let the sauce simmer for 2•3 minutes until slightly thickened.

7. Return the cooked chicken breasts to the skillet and spoon the lemon•caper sauce over the top. Serve the chicken piccata immediately, with lemon wedges on the side.

This chicken piccata is a great option for seniors on a renal diet for a few reasons:

- Chicken is a lean protein that's low in sodium and potassium
- The lemon•caper sauce is low in sodium, using just a small amount of chicken broth
- Capers add a nice briny flavor without much added salt

The bright, tangy sauce complements the tender chicken perfectly. Serve this dish with a side of roasted vegetables or a simple salad for a complete renal•friendly meal.

102. Mushroom risotto (low•fat cheese)

Ingredient:

- 1 tbsp olive oil
- 1 onion, finely chopped
- 2 cloves garlic, minced
- 8 oz (225g) mushrooms, sliced
- 1 cup (200g) arborio rice
- 1/2 cup (120ml) dry white wine
- 4 cups (1 liter) low•sodium vegetable or chicken broth, heated
- 1/2 cup (50g) low•fat grated parmesan cheese
- 2 tbsp low•fat cream cheese
- Salt and pepper to taste
- Chopped parsley for garnish (optional)

Instructions:

1. In a large saucepan, heat the olive oil over medium heat. Add the onion and sauté for 2•3 minutes until translucent.

2. Add the garlic and mushrooms and cook for 5 minutes, stirring occasionally, until the mushrooms are softened.

3. Add the arborio rice and stir to coat with the oil. Pour in the white wine and cook, stirring constantly, until the wine is absorbed.

4. Add the hot broth 1/2 cup at a time, stirring constantly, until the rice is tender and has a creamy consistency, about 18•20 minutes total.

5. Remove from heat and stir in the parmesan cheese and cream cheese until well combined. Season with salt and pepper to taste.

6. Serve the mushroom risotto immediately, garnished with chopped parsley if desired.

The low•fat cheeses help keep this risotto creamy without adding too much fat. Enjoy!

103. Zucchini noodles with marinara sauce

Ingredient:

- 3 medium zucchini, spiralized or julienned into noodles
- 1 tbsp olive oil
- 1 onion, diced
- 3 cloves garlic, minced
- 1 (14 oz) can low•sodium diced tomatoes
- 2 tbsp tomato paste
- 1 tsp dried oregano
- 1/4 tsp red pepper flakes (optional)
- Salt and pepper to taste
- Chopped fresh basil for garnish (optional)

Instructions:

1. Using a spiralizer or julienne peeler, cut the zucchini into long, thin noodles. Set aside.

2. In a large skillet, heat the olive oil over medium heat. Add the diced onion and sauté for 5 minutes until translucent.

3. Add the minced garlic and cook for 1 minute more, until fragrant.

4. Stir in the can of low•sodium diced tomatoes, tomato paste, oregano, and red pepper flakes (if using). Season with a pinch of salt and pepper.

5. Bring the marinara sauce to a simmer and let it cook for 5•7 minutes, stirring occasionally, until thickened slightly.

6. Add the zucchini noodles to the skillet and toss to coat them in the sauce. Cook for 2•3 minutes, just until the zucchini is tender.

7. Remove from heat and serve the zucchini noodles with marinara immediately, garnished with chopped fresh basil if desired.

The spiralized zucchini noodles provide a pasta•like texture without the carbs and sodium of traditional pasta. Feel free to adjust the spices or add any other low•potassium veggies to the marinara sauce.

Enjoy this simple yet flavorful zucchini noodle dish! Let me know if you need any other renal•friendly recipe ideas.

104. Spinach and ricotta stuffed shells

Ingredient:

- 12 jumbo pasta shells
- 1 cup part•skim ricotta cheese
- 1 cup chopped fresh spinach, stems removed
- 1/4 cup grated Parmesan cheese
- 1 egg, lightly beaten
- 1/4 tsp garlic powder
- 1/4 tsp dried oregano
- 1/4 tsp salt
- 1/8 tsp black pepper
- 1 cup low•sodium marinara sauce

Instructions:

1. Preheat oven to 375°F.

2. Cook the pasta shells according to package instructions until al dente. Drain and set aside.

3. In a medium bowl, mix together the ricotta cheese, spinach, Parmesan, egg, garlic powder, oregano, salt, and pepper until well combined.

4. Stuff each cooked pasta shell with about 2•3 tablespoons of the ricotta•spinach mixture.

5. Spread 1/2 cup of the low•sodium marinara sauce in the bottom of a baking dish. Arrange the stuffed shells in a single layer on top of the sauce.

6. Cover the dish with foil and bake for 20•25 minutes, until the shells are heated through.

7. Remove the foil and serve the stuffed shells warm, with the remaining marinara sauce spooned over the top.

This recipe is kidney•friendly as it is low in sodium and protein. The ricotta and spinach provide nutrients without being too high in phosphorus or potassium, which are important considerations for a renal diet. The low•sodium marinara sauce also helps keep the sodium content in check.

105. Polenta with grilled vegetables

Ingredient:

• 1 cup polenta
• 4 cups low•sodium vegetable or chicken broth
• 1 tbsp olive oil
• 1 zucchini, sliced into 1/2•inch rounds
• 1 yellow squash, sliced into 1/2•inch rounds
• 1 red bell pepper, sliced into strips
• 1 red onion, sliced into 1/2•inch rings
• 2 tbsp balsamic vinegar
• 1 tsp dried oregano
• Salt and pepper to taste
• Grated Parmesan cheese (optional)

Instructions:

1. In a medium saucepan, bring the broth to a boil over high heat. Slowly whisk in the polenta, reduce heat to low, and cook, stirring frequently, until the polenta is thick and creamy, about 15•20 minutes. Season with salt and pepper to taste.

2. Preheat grill or grill pan to medium•high heat.

3. In a large bowl, toss the sliced zucchini, yellow squash, bell pepper, and onion with the olive oil, balsamic vinegar, and oregano. Season with salt and pepper.

4. Grill the vegetables for 3•5 minutes per side, or until they are tender and lightly charred.

5. Spoon the hot polenta into bowls or plates. Top with the grilled vegetables, arranging them in an attractive pattern.

6. If desired, sprinkle the polenta and vegetables with grated Parmesan cheese.

7. Serve the polenta with grilled vegetables immediately, while hot.

This dish is a great way to enjoy the flavors of grilled vegetables paired with creamy, comforting polenta. The low•sodium broth and lack of added salt make it a healthier option. Feel free to use any combination of your favorite grilled vegetables.

Enjoy this delicious and nutritious polenta with grilled vegetables!

106. BBQ chicken breast (homemade sauce, low·sodium)

Ingredient:

For the BBQ Sauce:
- 1 cup no·salt·added tomato sauce
- 2 tbsp apple cider vinegar
- 1 tbsp Dijon mustard
- 1 tbsp honey
- 1 tsp smoked paprika
- 1/2 tsp garlic powder
- 1/4 tsp ground black pepper

For the Chicken:
- 4 boneless, skinless chicken breasts
- 1 tbsp olive oil
- Salt and pepper to taste

Instructions:

1. Make the BBQ Sauce:
- In a small saucepan, combine all the BBQ sauce ingredients. Whisk well to combine.
- Bring the sauce to a simmer over medium heat, then reduce heat to low and let it simmer for 10·15 minutes, stirring occasionally, until thickened slightly.
- Remove from heat and set aside.

2. Prepare the Chicken:
- Preheat grill or grill pan to medium·high heat.
- Rub the chicken breasts all over with the olive oil and season with salt and pepper.
- Grill the chicken for 5·7 minutes per side, or until cooked through and no longer pink in the center.

3. Baste and Finish:
- During the last 2·3 minutes of grilling, brush the chicken breasts generously with the homemade BBQ sauce, turning to coat both sides.
- Continue grilling until the sauce is caramelized and the chicken is cooked through.

4. Serve:
- Transfer the BBQ chicken breasts to a serving plate.
- Drizzle any remaining BBQ sauce over the top.
- Serve the BBQ chicken immediately, while hot.

The homemade low·sodium BBQ sauce is the star of this dish, providing a flavorful and healthier alternative to store·bought sauces. Pair the BBQ chicken with roasted vegetables or a fresh salad for a complete meal.

107. Grilled vegetable skewers

Ingredient:

- 1 zucchini, cut into 1•inch pieces
- 1 yellow squash, cut into 1•inch pieces
- 1 red bell pepper, cut into 1•inch pieces
- 1 yellow onion, cut into 1•inch pieces
- 8 oz mushrooms, halved
- 2 tbsp olive oil
- 1 tsp dried oregano
- 1 tsp dried basil
- 1/2 tsp garlic powder
- Salt and pepper to taste
- Wooden or metal skewers

Instructions:

1. Preheat grill to medium•high heat.

2. In a large bowl, toss the chopped vegetables with the olive oil, oregano, basil, garlic powder, salt, and pepper until evenly coated.

3. Thread the vegetables onto the skewers, alternating the different types.

4. Grill the vegetable skewers for 12•15 minutes, turning occasionally, until the vegetables are tender and lightly charred.

5. Serve the grilled vegetable skewers hot, as a main dish or side.

Tips:
- Soak wooden skewers in water for 30 minutes before using to prevent them from burning.
- You can use any combination of your favorite vegetables, such as eggplant, cherry tomatoes, asparagus, etc.
- Brush the skewers with a bit of olive oil or balsamic glaze before serving for extra flavor.
- Serve with a side of grilled bread or over a bed of quinoa or rice for a more substantial meal.

Enjoy these healthy and flavorful grilled vegetable skewers!

108. Turkey burgers with low•sodium condiments

Ingredient:

• 1 lb ground turkey
• 1/4 cup whole wheat breadcrumbs
• 1 egg, lightly beaten
• 1 tbsp Dijon mustard
• 1 tsp dried oregano
• 1/2 tsp garlic powder
• 1/4 tsp black pepper
• 4 whole wheat burger buns
• Low•sodium condiments:
  • Low•sodium ketchup
  • Low•sodium mustard
  • Sliced tomatoes
  • Lettuce leaves
  • Sliced onion (optional)

Instructions:

1. In a large bowl, combine the ground turkey, breadcrumbs, egg, Dijon mustard, oregano, garlic powder, and black pepper. Mix well until all the ingredients are evenly distributed.

2. Divide the turkey mixture into 4 equal portions and shape them into patties, about 4•5 inches wide and 1/2 inch thick.

3. Preheat a grill or grill pan to medium•high heat. Lightly oil the grill grates or pan to prevent the burgers from sticking.

4. Grill the turkey burgers for 4•5 minutes per side, or until they are cooked through and reach an internal temperature of 165°F.

5. Toast the whole wheat burger buns on the grill for 1•2 minutes, until lightly golden.

6. Assemble the burgers by placing a turkey patty on each bun. Top with the low•sodium condiments of your choice, such as low•sodium ketchup, low•sodium mustard, sliced tomatoes, lettuce leaves, and sliced onion (if using). Serve the turkey burgers immediately, while hot.

The use of low•sodium condiments helps keep the overall sodium content of this dish lower, making it a healthier option for those on a low•sodium diet. The whole wheat buns and breadcrumbs also add fiber and nutrients

109. Grilled portobello mushrooms with balsamic glaze

Ingredient:

- 4 large portobello mushroom caps, stems removed
- 2 tbsp olive oil
- 2 tbsp balsamic vinegar
- 2 tbsp brown sugar
- 1 tsp garlic powder
- 1/2 tsp dried thyme
- Salt and pepper to taste

For the Balsamic Glaze:
- 1/2 cup balsamic vinegar
- 2 tbsp brown sugar

Instructions:

1. Make the balsamic glaze: In a small saucepan, combine the 1/2 cup balsamic vinegar and 2 tbsp brown sugar. Bring to a simmer over medium heat, stirring occasionally, until the mixture has reduced by half and thickened to a glaze•like consistency, about 10•15 minutes. Remove from heat and set aside.

2. Preheat grill or grill pan to medium•high heat.

3. In a shallow dish, whisk together the 2 tbsp olive oil, 2 tbsp balsamic vinegar, 2 tbsp brown sugar, garlic powder, dried thyme, salt, and pepper.

4. Add the portobello mushroom caps to the marinade and turn to coat both sides.

5. Grill the marinated mushrooms for 4•5 minutes per side, until tender and lightly charred.

6. Transfer the grilled mushrooms to a serving plate and drizzle the balsamic glaze over the top.

7. Serve the grilled portobello mushrooms immediately, while hot.

The balsamic glaze adds a sweet and tangy flavor that complements the savory mushrooms perfectly. This makes a great main dish or side for a summer grilling menu.

110. BBQ shrimp skewers

Ingredient:

• 1 lb large shrimp, peeled and deveined
• 2 tbsp olive oil
• 2 tbsp brown sugar
• 2 tbsp Worcestershire sauce
• 1 tbsp lemon juice
• 1 tsp smoked paprika
• 1/2 tsp garlic powder
• 1/4 tsp cayenne pepper (optional, for spice)
• Salt and pepper to taste
• Wooden or metal skewers

Instructions:

1. In a medium bowl, combine the olive oil, brown sugar, Worcestershire sauce, lemon juice, smoked paprika, garlic powder, and cayenne pepper (if using). Season with salt and pepper.

2. Add the shrimp to the marinade and toss to coat evenly. Cover and refrigerate for 30 minutes to 1 hour.

3. Preheat grill or grill pan to medium•high heat.

4. Thread the marinated shrimp onto the skewers, leaving a little space between each shrimp.

5. Grill the shrimp skewers for 2•3 minutes per side, or until the shrimp are opaque and cooked through.

6. Serve the BBQ shrimp skewers immediately, while hot.

Tips:
• Soak wooden skewers in water for 30 minutes before using to prevent them from burning.
• You can use a combination of different types of shrimp, such as jumbo, tiger, or even small shrimp.
• Adjust the amount of cayenne pepper to your desired level of spiciness.
• Serve the BBQ shrimp skewers with grilled vegetables, rice, or a fresh salad for a complete meal.

As we conclude the **"Renal Diet Cookbook for Seniors Over 60: 110+ Recipes – A Comprehensive Guide to Managing Renal Health,"** we hope this journey through kidney-friendly cuisine has been both enlightening and enriching for you.

Throughout this cookbook, our aim has been to provide not just recipes, but a comprehensive resource to support your renal health goals. We understand the challenges and complexities that come with managing kidney health, especially as we age. By focusing on nutrient-rich ingredients, portion control, and mindful meal planning, we have strived to make it easier for you to enjoy delicious meals while supporting your kidneys.

We've explored a variety of flavors and cooking techniques, from comforting soups and stews to vibrant salads and satisfying main dishes, ensuring there is something to suit every palate and preference. Each recipe has been designed with your health in mind, incorporating ingredients that are gentle on the kidneys yet bursting with flavor.

Beyond recipes, this book has served as a guide, equipping you with essential knowledge about renal health, dietary guidelines, and practical tips for navigating grocery aisles and meal preparation. We hope you've found value in understanding how different nutrients impact kidney function and how to make informed choices that promote your well-being.

As you continue on your journey to maintain or improve your renal health, remember that small changes can make a significant difference. Whether you are following this diet for preventive measures or managing kidney disease, your dedication to your health is commendable. Consistency and balance are key, and this cookbook is here to support you every step of the way.

We encourage you to experiment with the recipes, adapt them to your taste preferences, and continue exploring new ways to nourish yourself while caring for your kidneys. By making mindful choices and enjoying meals that are both nutritious and delicious, you are taking proactive steps toward a healthier future.

Thank you for choosing this cookbook as your companion in your journey toward better kidney health. We wish you continued success and wellness in all your culinary adventures and beyond.

With warmest regards,

Daisy Robinson